HEAD AND NECK INJURIES IN SPORTS

HEAD AND NECK INJURIES
IN SPORTS

By

STEPHEN E. REID, M.S., M.D.

Vice Chairman, Department of Surgery
Evanston Hospital
Evanston, Illinois

Professor of Surgery
Northwestern University Medical School
Chicago, Illinois

and

STEPHEN E. REID, JR., M.D.

Department of Surgical Oncology
Roswell Park Memorial Institute
Buffalo, New York

With Contributions by

Stephen E. Long, B.S., M.S.

and

Gil Raviv, M.S.

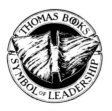

C H A R L E S C T H O M A S • P U B L I S H E R
Springfield • Illinois • U.S.A.

Published and Distributed Throughout the World by

CHARLES C THOMAS • PUBLISHER

2600 South First Street

Springfield, Illinois 62717

© *1984 by* CHARLES C THOMAS • PUBLISHER

ISBN 0-398-04974-2

Library of Congress Catalog Card Number: 83-24294

With THOMAS BOOKS *careful attention is given to all details of manufacturing and
design. It is the Publisher's desire to present books that are satisfactory as to their physical
qualities and artistic possibilities and appropriate for their particular use.* THOMAS
BOOKS *will be true to those laws of quality that assure a good name and good will.*

Printed in the United States of America
Q–R–3

Library of Congress Cataloging in Publication Data

Reid, Stephen E. (Stephen Emmett), 1914–
    Head and neck injuries in sports.

    Bibliography: p.
    Includes index.
    1. Head—Wounds and injuries.   2. Neck—Wounds and
injuries.   3. First aid in illness and injury.   4. Sports
—Accidents and injuries.   I. Reid, Stephen E.   II. Title.
[DNLM: 1. Athletic injuries—Therapy.   2. Head injuries—
Therapy.   3. Neck—Injuries.   4. First aid. WA 292 R358h]
RD521.R454   1984   617'.51044   83-24294
ISBN 0-398-04974-2

To our wife and mother, Grace B. Reid.

PREFACE

The senior author, with over thirty years' experience as the team physician for Northwestern University's athletic teams, the doctor for the Tribune All-Star Games, and All-American guard on the Northwestern University Big Ten Championship football team, has observed many changes in both the sports themselves and in the athletes participating in these sports. As spectator sports have grown in popularity over the years, the demand for continual improvement in the areas of equipment, player conditioning, coaching, officiating, and team medical personnel has similarly increased. The strides made have been significant, but the incidence of sports-related injuries still remains a very real problem.

Head and neck injuries have the potential for the most serious consequences of any sports-related injury. The radio-telemetry data obtained during fifteen football seasons at Northwestern University has given us tremendous insight into the causes of head and neck injuries. In many instances, such injuries can be avoided entirely if the coaches and players understand the mechanisms of injury and the methods that can be utilized to prevent such injury. When an injury does occur, however, it is crucial that it be immediately and correctly identified and treated, with a specific and intensive rehabilitation program initiated after healing has occurred.

This book is directed toward team physicians, coaches, trainers, athletic officials, and athletes, all of whom must work together to prevent sports-related injuries and to manage those injuries that do occur. This treatise is concerned with on-the-spot recognition of head and neck injuries, first-aid treatment, and disposition of the injured athlete.

S.E.R.
S.E.R. Jr.

ACKNOWLEDGMENTS

A book such as this cannot be written without the help of many individuals. We would like to express our gratitude to Michael W. Louis, the W. W. Grainger Foundation, Inc., the Sports Foundation, Inc., the Evanston Hospital, and the Northwestern University Medical School for their financial support of our research. In addition, we are deeply indebted to a dedicated group of people who gave both time and encouragement to this project. They include first and foremost Doctor Herbert Epstein; also, Doctor Joseph Tarkington, Doctor Michael Mikhael, George Reifenach, John Reid, John Danielson, Coaches Ara Parseghian and Alex Agase, and the Northwestern University Athletic Department.

Our research would not have been possible without the participation of the Northwestern University varsity football players who agreed to wear the telemetry equipment during each game of the season. These players, over the fifteen-year period during which we collected our data, include: Bill Swingle, Steve Murphy, Woody Campbell, Bill Galler, Mike Varty, Al Draper, Joe Paternchak, Al Benz, Jack Durning, John Voorhees, Bob Olson, Scott Duncan, Greg Stanley, and Steve Ananen. During this time, the biomedical engineering expertise was provided by Thomas O'Dea, M. L. Petrovick, and Nijas Zenkich.

Finally, as we began to write up the results of our research, we were helped enormously by Morvin Mellor and his staff of the Audio-Visual Department and by Rose Slowinski, head librarian of the Webster Medical Library at the Evanston Hospital, and by June Hill Pedigo, who drew all of the illustrations in the book. We want to thank Kate Bauman, who typed the early portions of the manuscript. The major portion of the text was typed by Laura Balin. We are very grateful to her for her time and patience in typing the many revisions and checking the bibliography and illustrations. Lastly, we would like to thank Michele Grygotis for her excellent editorial assistance of the entire book.

CONTENTS

HEAD AND NECK INJURIES IN SPORTS

Chapter 1

THE PROBLEM OF
HEAD AND NECK INJURIES IN SPORTS

When one speaks of head and neck injuries, the sports most commonly involved are football, wrestling, aquatic diving, and trampoline. The game of football has been played in many parts of the world and has survived from ancient times. Association football, or soccer, is played with a round ball that must always be kicked, never carried. Rugby, another variation of football, is played with an oval ball that may either be carried or kicked but not passed forward. American football is a direct descendant of British rugby and is also played with an oval ball, but in this variation the ball may be kicked, passed, or carried in any direction. In Great Britain, rugby was considered a diversion for youths of the lower classes. At the turn of the nineteenth century, public schools brought these youths together to participate in the sport, but university undergraduates considered the game boisterous and undignified for scholarly young gentlemen. At about this time, American football was taken up by students in both schools and colleges. American football today has evolved from many years of playing under various sectional rules into a precise sport.

Football attracts a certain type of individual, someone who cannot be satisfied with any other sport. The participants are vigorous young men requiring a body-contact sport to satisfy their needs. Football directs their energy into an activity where similar individuals can complete in a supervised fashion without the risk of doing serious injury to the less physically powerful. In addition, football can motivate a young person to continue his education through the program of college athletic scholarships. The result is that many of these athletes have completed their college educations and have been prepared for worthwhile careers. Since many of these athletes come from families of limited means, these young men would be unable to attend college were it not for athletic scholarships. Football, therefore, not only provides an acceptable outlet for physical aggression, but it also provides educational opportunities to athletes who qualify for college athletic scholarships.

Football is enjoyed by spectators of all ages and both sexes. Television has certainly stimulated this interest, to the degree that football now occupies

3

the number-one position in sports popularity today. Newspapers and sports-casters, aware of the interest that the public has in sports and football in particular, allot increasing time and space to this type of coverage. An article written in the *Wall Street Journal* by Frederick C. Klein, September 5, 1974, is entitled "Is College Football Out of Control?" This article pointed out that the American Broadcasting Company (ABC) is paying $16 million for the rights to show this year's college games and the degree to which college sports have dived into the general scramble for the American entertainment dollar. This issue has troubled educators for years, but trustees tend not to be the agents of change. With the current stress on physical fitness, it seems likely that interest in sports will continue to increase and, therefore, work-able solutions to the problems associated with football will have to be found, since outlawing the sport appears to be an untenable alternative.

When one considers the problems associated with football, perhaps the most significant one that comes to mind is that of football-related injuries. This chapter will attempt to examine the problem and pose solutions to it. Any sport that involves the vigorous body contact that football does would be expected to cause some injuries. Minor injuries are inherent to the game and are not included in this discussion. Even the injury that puts the player out of the game or prevents him from playing the sport again, while not causing permanent damage, cannot be included in these statistics. Admittedly, efforts should be made to eliminate *all* injuries, but it is the injuries that result in fatalities or severe non-fatal injuries that concern us here. Included in this latter group are those injuries that may not be considered serious but which have major sequelae, such as post-traumatic epilepsy.

Statistics on fatalities have been compiled annually since 1931 by the American Football Coaches Association, and this source is to be commended for its thorough reporting of deaths due to football.[1] It has been estimated that about 90 percent of football-related deaths are due to head and neck injuries.[12] These figures, however, do not include those serious injuries that result in permanent disability, and there has been no extensive collection of data on these types of injuries until recently. For example, twelve severe head and neck injuries occurred in the states of Pennsylvania and New Jersey in 1975; eight of these injuries resulted in quadriparesis but none could be included in fatality statistics. The most complete survey of such statistics was reported by the National Football Head and Neck Injury Registry in 1978.[12] This data was compared to the figures reported by Schneider[8] and the National Athletic Injury/Illness Reporting System (NAIRS),[3] and these reports indicated a decrease in the incidence of serious head injuries, with a corresponding increase in the incidence of serious neck injuries. In another series of 1,600 patients admitted to the hospital, 152 (9.5%) suffered cervical cord damage while participating in recreational athletics. Fifty-five percent occurred while diving, while only 11 percent sustained their injuries in football.[9]

When we speak of football-related injuries that result in permanent disability, we are talking of injuries to the head and neck.[2] Injuries to the bony skull alone are not considered to be serious injuries, and the incidence of skull fractures are extremely rare. Brain injury, categorized as concussion, is defined as *a usually temporary loss of consciousness in the post-traumatic state, accompanied by little, if any, gross brain damage.* There are, however, degress of severity of concussion, depending upon the length of unconsciousness and the extent of post-traumatic memory loss.[11] The most serious head injuries are those that result in contusions or lacerations in the brain substance or which cause hemorrhaging within or around the brain. The hemorrhage causes increased pressure within the skull, which can be fatal if this pressure is not immediately released surgically. Post-traumatic epilepsy can result from concussion and usually begins within two years of head injury. The incidence of epilepsy following head injury is approximately 3 percent, and electroencephalograms generally reveal brain damage in these cases.[5,7,13]

Football-related injuries to the cervical spine are classified as serious injuries, and properly so. These neck injuries are divided into two groups: (1) upper cervical spine (C_1 through C_3) and (2) lower cervical spine (C_4 through C_7). Injuries to the upper cervical spine are very uncommon in football; the most common lower cervical spine injury involves the C_5 to C_6 level. This injury usually results from a blow to the top of the helmet caused by a player being struck with his head in a flexed position. In this position the entire force is borne by the bony structure of the neck, and a fracture dislocation occurs. A transection of the spinal cord occurs, with complete and permanent paralysis below this level. An athlete can receive this injury when he resorts to "spearing" to intimidate an opponent or when he ducks his head in an attempt to avoid injury. This injury uncommonly occurs with severe hyperextension of the neck, usually as a component of a whiplash effect, when a blow is delivered at some unguarded moment. A common football injury is the so-called nerve pinch. This is actually an injury to the brachial plexus and can result in a contusion of the axillary nerve from a direct blow to the top of the shoulder and base of the neck, or due to a stretch of the plexus from a blow directed to the side of the head. Although muscle contusion and ligament strain may accompany this lesion, sensory loss in the skin overlying the deltoid muscle, with some loss of deltoid function, is commonly present. While this injury is not inherently dangerous, it does present a problem for the team physician, since it may be difficult to differentiate it from the serious cervical cord lesion. The arm on the affected side hangs limply by the side, and the athlete complains of intense burning pain radiating from the root of the neck, out over the shoulder, and down the arm. This usually lasts for several minutes and gradually disappears. Another type of brachial plexus injury involves a contusion of the nerve root at the intervertebral foramen, resulting from a blow to the opposite side of the head, which then causes a lateral flexion of the cervical spine. Radiating pain in this type of injury is more intense than in the more peripheral brachial plexus injury. An athlete some years ago incurred repeated nerve root injury that caused nearly complete paralysis and atrophy of the triceps muscle. His neck was explored, and marked scarring was found at the intervertebral foramen.

When a catastrophic injury occurs on the football field, the blame for this injury must be shared. The helmet receives the brunt of the attack; its protective mechanism is blamed as being too rigid, not rigid enough, cut too low over the neck, or not equipped with an outer cushion to avoid such an injury. The face mask is also blamed. The charge is made that because it affords so much protection, the athlete has no fear and uses his head as a battering ram in spearing. It is also charged that the face mask offers a convenient handle to grasp, causing undue strain to be put on the player's neck when his head is violently jerked. The coach is blamed for his "win-at-all-costs" attitude and for teaching head-on and butt blocking. The tackler who aims his shoulder at an elusive ball carrier is more likely to miss the tackle than if he aimed his head at the center of the ball carrier's body. It is for this reason that the athlete is taught to stick his head at the center of the ball carrier's body, at the numbers on the player's jersey. Although this approach is a good way to bring the ball carrier down, it may put the head of the tackler in jeopardy of the full force of the opponent or, even worse, the pumping action of the ball carrier's knees. These same principles apply to the blocker who practices butt blocking. In some instances, the coach may develop the "killer instinct" in his players to a dangerous degree in order to intimidate the opponent. The coach may also be accused of improper selection of players or of inadequately conditioning his team. He may be blamed for overworking the players to the point of fatigue or for allowing partially disabled players to continue in the game. The football rules committee also receives a share of the blame, and this group has been criticized for permitting dangerous acts to occur on the playing field, such as the so-called "chop block" used by interior linemen. The game officials must be held responsible for the safe conduct of the game, and they are often blamed for their laissez-faire attitude. As former players themselves, they seem to believe that the game should be played with a minimum of interference, since too many penalties spoil the spectacle. School officials are open to the criticism that they pay too little attention to the sport and place unqualified people in charge of the games. Another criticism is that medical care to injured players is inadequate, sometimes provided by the coach or similarly unqualified person. Since few high school teams have designated team physicians, it is not uncommon for any doctor who happens to be present at a game to be called upon in the event of an injury on the field: a very unsatisfactory arrangement.

The concern over serious football-related injuries is justified, but correcting the existing deficiencies that contribute to these injuries is a difficult task. Nonetheless, assessment of these deficiencies is necessary, and potential solutions to the problem of football injuries must be carefully examined.[4,6,10]

One of the problems in the evaluation of head and neck injuries as they relate to the football helmet is that the helmet is tested in simulated conditions in the laboratory. These tests, although establishing the strength of the helmet material, in no way demonstrate the tolerance levels of the human head and neck. Moreover, there is no information available on the cumulative effects on the brain to repeated, medium-intensity blows. A thorough discussion of the football helmet will take place in Chapter 2.

The coach and the players themselves play crucial roles in the prevention of football-related injuries. With regard to the role of the coach, he must temper his desire to win with his concern for player safety, and his team must understand this. The coach must impress upon the players the dangers of maneuvers such as head-on tackling and butt blocking. Several years ago, Northwestern had a rash of brachial plexus injuries. When Coach Parseghian realized that this was the result of the player driving his head into an opponent in blocking and tackling, he changed his coaching techniques and the incidence of this injury fell dramatically. Increasing neck muscle conditioning or shifting the player who incurs recurrent injury to the other side of the line will also help to prevent these injuries. The coach must not allow an awkward boy with a long, thin neck to play football until he has developed sufficient strength and agility to protect himself from injury. Proper player conditioning must be a continual concern of a coach, who can share in the duty of conditioning drills with the team trainer. In addition, the coach must be aware of the role that player fatigue and partially disabled athletes play in football injuries. A fatigued or injured player is incapable of the quick maneuvers that can often avoid injury. The coach must recognize this and use his judgment to withdraw these players from the field regardless of the effect of such withdrawal on the outcome of the game.

The player himself must assume part of the responsibility for preventing injuries on the field. He must also recognize the importance of conditioning and continually inspect and maintain his own equipment. The player needs to realize, however, that he cannot rely solely on his equipment for protection. As was previously mentioned, too often players become overconfident about the protective qualities of their equipment, particularly the helmet, which results in dangerous risk-taking on the field. Players must understand that recklessness has no place on the football field, and the player who believes that it does will soon discover that he has exceeded his body's tolerance to impact. A professional player a few years ago believed that he was too tough to be injured, regardless of the recklessness with which he played. After bending several face masks, he was finally fitted with a much more rigid device, only to go on to distort this mask to such a degree that a hacksaw was required to cut it off in order to remove the helmet. He subsequently suffered a cervical fracture and was unable to play the game again. Finally, the player must accept some responsibility for protecting his fellow team members, and even the opposing team players, from injury. To use the face mask as an example again, it was designed to prevent facial and oral injuries, but it is frequently used as a handle for the opposing player to grasp and violently jerk. This can result in cervical spine injury and brain damage caused by the torsion of the head when it is pulled. Clearly, then, the athlete himself can play a very active role in preventing injuries during the game, both to himself and to other players on the field.

It is the responsibility of the officials of the game of football to make changes in the rules of the game when it becomes obvious that existing rules contribute to or fail to prevent injury. Many rule changes are already in effect, but more changes need to be made. For example, clipping downfield has been outlawed for several years, since a player is extremely vulnerable to injury when an opponent strikes from the player's blind side. Clipping within three yards of the line of scrimmage was permissible, however, until it became evident that the ends were being injured by the so-called "crack-back-block," which actually was a clip. The rules committee, recognizing this, then outlawed clipping at the extreme ends of the line of scrimmage. Presently, clipping is being done in the interior of the line, and this chop block is very harmful to the defensive linesman's knees. This is unquestionably a dangerous play that has recently been outlawed. During the actual playing of the game, the officials need to keep a vigilant watch and penalize those procedures, such as grabbing the face mask, which can lead to injuries. Rule changes and rule enforcement are essential to the prevention of injuries and should not be considered as distractions from the spectacle of the sport.

A certified team trainer is an integral part of the football program. He can be instrumental in preventing injuries or in minimizing their severity, for he has been trained to recognize potentially serious injuries, understands proper taping techniques to support injured parts, can teach conditioning exercises, and has received instruction in the rehabilitation of the injured athlete. The trainer must, however, work in conjunction with the team physician, who must make the final decision concerning all injuries, minor or major in nature. Unfortunately, however, many schools do not have a designated team doctor, and this is a deficiency that should be remedied. The team physician must take an active role in preventing and/or minimizing player injuries, and this begins with getting well acquainted with every player on the team. Any team doctor knows that there are some players who magnify the slightest injury, while there are others who refuse to acknowledge an injury or who minimize its seriousness. Only by knowing each player well and having a familiarity with the medical history of each member of the team can the physician accurately assess each athlete's playing condition and diagnose injuries that do occur.

Finally, spectators, in their enthusiasm to see their team win, must keep in mind the importance of player safety. Officials who call penalties on plays that have the potential for causing injuries should not be harassed by the fans, nor should the coaches who refuse to play by the "win-no-matter-what" philosophy. Fans who recognize the importance of player safety will do much to reinforce this concept in the minds of the officials, coaches, and players.

It becomes obvious, then, that the responsibility for preventing football-related injuries must be shared among everyone concerned with the game, from the companies who design football equipment down to the fans who attend the game. The incidence of serious injuries can be reduced only if each group assumes its proper responsibility for ensuring player safety. Once this happens, then one of the biggest objections to the sport—that it is too dangerous—can be proven groundless.

REFERENCES

1. Blythe, C. S., and Arnold, D. C.: Forty-Seventh Annual Survey of Football Fatalities: 1931–1978. Paper presented at American Football Coaches Association, National Collegiate Athletic Association and the National Federation of State High Schools Association, Feb., 1979.
2. Clark, K. S.: A survey of sports-related spinal cord injuries in schools and colleges. *J Safety Res, 9:*140, 1977.
3. Clark, K. S., and Powell, J. W.: Football helmets and neurotrauma: an epidemiological overview of three seasons. *Med & Sci in Sports, 11:*138, 1979.
4. Dinman, B.: The reality and acceptance of risk. *JAMA, 244:*1226, 1980.
5. Hendrix, E. B., and Harris, L.: Post-traumatic epilepsy in children. *Engl J Trauma, 8:*547, 1968.
6. Maroon, J. C., and Healion, T.: Head and neck injuries in football. *J Indiana State Med Assn, 63:*225, 1970.
7. Payor, H., Loga, M., and Berard-Badies, M.: The pathology of posttraumatic epilepsy. *Engl Epilepsia,* Amsterdam, March, 1970.
8. Schneider, R. D.: *Head and Neck Injuries in Football: Mechanisms, Treatment and Prevention.* Baltimore, Williams and Wilkins, 1973.
9. Shields, C. L., Fox, J. M., and Stouffer, E.: Cervical cord injuries in sports. *The Physician & Sports Med,* p. 71, Sept., 1978.
10. Straub, W. F., and Davis, S. W.: Personality traits of college football players who participate at different levels of competition. *Med & Sci in Sports, 3:*39, 1971.
11. Subcommittee on Classification of Sports Injuries, Committee on Medical Aspects of Sports of AMA: Cerebral Concussion, Acute First, Second and Third Degree. *Standard Nomenclature of Athletic Injuries,* Vol. 20, 1966.
12. Torg, J. S., Truex, R., Quedenfield, T. C., et al: The national football head and neck injury registry: report and conclusions. *JAMA, 241:*1477, 1979 (see Chapter 12).
13. Walker, A. E.: Post-traumatic epilepsy: mechanism of cerebral trauma. In Youmans, J. (Ed.): *Neurologic Surgery.* Philadelphia, Saunders, 1973, Vol. 2, pp. 936–949.

Chapter 2

PROTECTIVE EQUIPMENT

The function of the helmet is to provide protection from injury to the integument of the head, including superficial wounds to the scalp and the ears. The headgear must protect the bony housing of the brain from fracture while also providing a means of absorbing the shock to the brain resulting from blows of low, medium, and high intensity. Clearly, in order to design an effective helmet, a knowledge of the tolerance of the brain to impact is essential. Blows of low intensity will cause discomfort when the helmet is designed to absorb only high-intensity impacts; in fact, the effect on the wearer would be the same if no protection were worn. Medium-intensity blows must be cushioned because of their cumulative effect upon the brain, and it is necessary to know the intensity of high-impact blows in order to provide adequate protection against them. The intensity and character of impacts vary with the sport, from the single, high-intensity blow typical of baseball, to the varied nature of the impact in hockey, and finally to the most complicated impacts encountered in football. The football helmet has drawn the most attention and will be discussed in detail. Unlike the crash helmet, a football helmet must be designed to withstand multiple blows. Therefore, it should be made of a material that will protect the head from one impact and then be immediately ready to protect against additional impacts. Because the greatest protection a player has is his own ability to avoid injury and since this ability is dependent upon the player having a full field of vision and hearing, the helmet shell must be designed so as not to reduce a player's peripheral vision or his hearing without compromising protection.[7] All of these specifications must be incorporated into a helmet that will not be a burden to carry throughout a game.

The composition of the outer surface of the helmet has varied over the years to conform with the changing game. The earliest helmets were leather and appeared around 1909. They offered little protection for the head, although they did have extensions down over the ears for their protection. Gradually, the leather helmet was modified to offer greater protection to the head, and eventually, in the late 1930s, a sturdy, leather helmet with an inner felt lining was produced. While the early leather helmet merely protected the ears and surface of the head from abrasions and lacerations, it offered very little protection for the skull and brain. This latter leather helmet was moderately stiff and was reinforced with leather bands across the crown. Because of the irregular contour of this headgear, glancing blows could not slip off the surface but would stick to it, and this design modification subjected the head to torque and possible head and neck injuries. Additionally, these helmets made very little attempt to distribute the force of impact over a large area of the head, and they offered little protection against skull fracture, necessitating that the player rely more on his own concern for self-preservation to avoid injury than on the helmet for protection. The absence of the face mask on the helmet undoubtedly contributed to this attitude. Interestingly enough, the concept that the player must rely upon himself, and not his equipment, for protection proved remarkably effective in preventing head and neck injuries. Up until 1943, when it became mandatory for all players on the field to wear helmets, it was not unusual for a player to remove his helmet and continue to play. Despite this, very few bare-headed players incurred head or neck injuries.

The plastic helmet was first introduced in 1939, but World War II delayed its popularity until the late 1940s. Theoretically, the plastic shell would present an impregnable defense to all blows. It would cause an impact to be distributed over a wide area of the head, thereby reducing the force per square inch on the head and avoiding skull fracture. However, to accomplish this goal, the shell would have had to be so thick that its size and weight would have been unacceptable. These limitations on the size and weight of the shell have resulted in a deformation of the shell under high- and medium-intensity blows. When indentation occurs, the suspension system alone, with no padding, is insufficient to prevent the shell from bottoming, because the space between the shell is reduced by the indentation of the shell of the helmet. The plastic shell, however, does offer far greater resistance to deformation than the leather helmet did, demonstrating the principle of dissipation of energy. Attempts to use material other than plastic to make the shell more resistant to deformation have thus far been unsuccessful.

The football helmet must dissipate the energy of a blow according to two main principles: spreading the force in time and spreading the force in space. The exact principle that applies to any given situation depends on several variables, including the intensity of the blow received by the helmet and the age, size, and ability of the player, who can range from a grade school student to the professional athlete. When the momentum of the striking body is reduced over a prolonged period of time, the force is spread out in time, and when the force is applied over a large area of the head, the force per square inch is reduced and the force is spread out in space. An example of the concept of force distribution would be spikes on a golf shoe. These spikes could ruin a linoleum floor if a golfer walked over it, while no damage would occur if the golfer walked over it wearing street shoes. It is the concentrated weight of the golfer pressing down on the floor in the very small area occupied by the point of the golf cleat, therefore, that causes the damage. The principle of spreading the force of the impact over a large area of the head avoids skull fractures in this same manner. In addition, the suspension system stretches as the shell is pressed to the head. This stretch prolongs the stopping time of the blow and provides the "give" that absorbs the blow, just as the life net of the fireman stretches when a person jumps into it from a burning building (Fig. 2-1). The suspension system of the helmet, however, must be stiff enough so that the shell will not strike the head of the wearer, thereby causing injury. Such contact is referred to as "bottoming." A padded helmet can distribute the blow, but impact can only be absorbed in these areas where padding is present (Fig. 2-2). As the padding is compressed, energy is absorbed. The distance the padding is compressed is related to the stopping time of the blow. The resiliency of the padding is extremely important here because subsequent blows must be absorbed immediately following the initial impact. Rigid padding will prevent bottoming when a large force is applied, and when this padding is depressed, it will assume its original thickness immediately after impact without a restoring force that adds to the force of the impact. This additional force is the rebound effect as the head bounces away from the site of the blow. Rigid padding absorbs very little energy, while padding that is compressed over a longer period of time, returning to its former shape over a longer period, will absorb energy but is likely to cause bottoming. A combination of the principles of dissipation of energy have been incorporated into helmet designs for the purpose of increasing the energy absorption of blows of great intensity. The fact that compression of air occurs during blows of low intensity resulted in the incorporation of air cells in some brands of helmets as well as standard padding to absorb blows of great intensity, with the air cells considered to be the first line of defense (Fig. 2-3). Because fluid is less compressible than air, the so-called "water helmet" was developed as a more effective cushion against high-intensity impacts (Fig. 2-4). The fluid used was a type of antifreeze (ethyleneglycol), which would not freeze when the temperature dropped below the freezing point. Although this helmet did seem to provide the greatest protection against high-intensity impacts, fluid leaks from the compartments, coupled with the additional weight of the helmet due to the fluid, created problems. Some helmets were designed incorporating fluid sacs connected by communicating channels, which was based on the theory that a blow would cause fluid to escape from the compressed compartment into another through communicating channels. In application, however, the inertia of the fluid prevented the rapid flow of fluid during the short duration of impact.

Various impact-testing devices for helmets have been used. One method

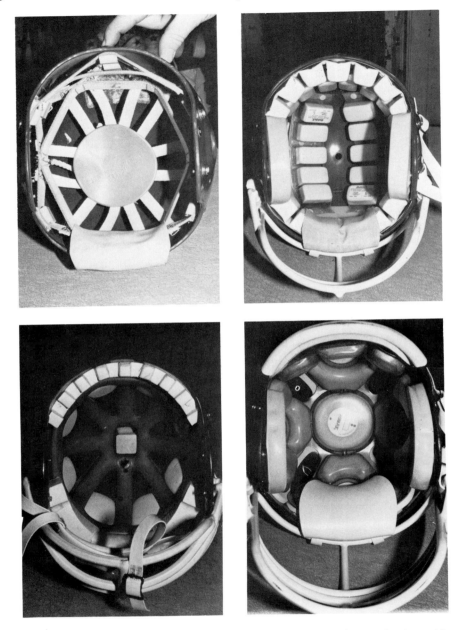

Figure 2-1. (Upper left) Suspension-type helmet shows simple interior mechanism with good ventilation.

Figure 2-2. (Upper right) Padded-type helmet shows padding that can be replaced when damaged.

Figure 2-3. (Lower left) Air helmet shows air cells that can be pumped with air for a snug fit.

Figure 2-4. (Lower right) Water helmet shows compartments that contain fluid.

of testing utilizes a pendulum in which a striker is swung into contact with the helmet. The more commonly used method for establishing standards for helmets, however, involves dropping a helmet onto a block. Accelerometers are secured at the center of gravity of the head form in the helmet in the latter test or are fixed to the striking bob in the former test (Fig. 2-5). With regard to the drop test, metal head forms were used for many years inside the helmets, which were then dropped onto cast iron platforms secured to concrete blocks. The drop test of the weighted helmet onto a cast-iron platform absorbed such little energy that the entire impact was accepted by the helmet, and the resultant deceleration was of such short duration that the velocity change, or foot pounds of energy, was a more meaningful measurement.[8] These precisely guided drops were repeated several times to ensure the durability of the various types of helmets. As time passed, helmet testing became more sophisticated. Metal head forms and wooden models were replaced by anthropomorphic head forms, which have response characteristics similar to heads of human cadavers.[6] The helmets are dropped from increasing heights until excessive accelerations are recorded or material failure occurs. Although this is indeed a comprehensive test of helmet material, the question still remains as to whether a living, human head protected by the helmet could tolerate the test impacts, even if the helmet material could, or whether a football player ever encounters such impacts. We do know, for instance, that helmet failure does occur on the football field without causing an injury to the player and that many players receive a concussion with no evidence of helmet failure (Fig. 2-6).

The National Operating Committee on Standards for Athletic Equipment, consisting of helmet manufacturers and distributors, attempted to answer the question of brain tolerance to impact with an acceleration-time tolerance curve.[6] This curve resulted from impact studies done with cadaveric and animal heads and was based on the assumption that the amount of force that will produce a linear skull fracture in a cadaver is equivalent to the force required to produce a moderate concussion in a living person. This very specific information was obtained through test studies of impacts of only the frontal aspect of the cadaveric skull onto a flat, hard surface in order to obtain the early part of the curve. The main portion of the curve was developed through animal experimentation.

While this curve plotted accelerations as a function of time, Gadd[3] plotted force against time and developed a severity index. By integrating test results and raising to the 2.5 exponent, a figure of 1,000 on this scale was determined to be the point of danger to life from frontal blows. These curves, as well as the J-tolerance value, which was developed by the Vienna Institute of Technology,[10] were based on specific conditions related to automobile-related impacts; they have little application to these impacts encountered on the

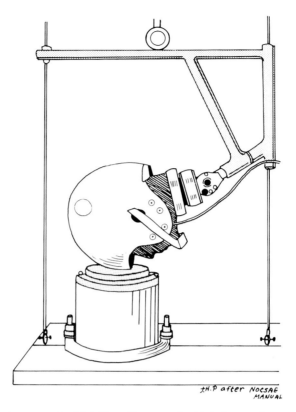

Figure 2-5. Helmet drop test. Artificial head is covered with helmet prior to testing and weighs approximately the same as a human head.

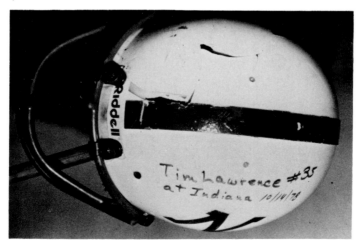

Figure 2-6. The player who cracked this helmet shell suffered no injury and only became aware that it was cracked when a teammate told him.

football field. A concussion tolerance curve is an attempt to bracket the upper limits of head acceleration that can be expected to occur on the football field. Unfortunately, the basic assumption that the force required to cause a linear skull fracture in a cadaveric head is equivalent to the force required to cause a moderate concussion in a living person is not supported by evidence.[4] There is very little relationship between skull fracture and the development of a cerebral dysfunction, concussion, or brain damage.[11] Furthermore, skull fractures are very uncommon in football, while the incidence of concussion is very significant. This curve, furthermore, applies only to the very specific conditions under which this data was collected and it has little application where other conditions prevail. An example of how impact data vary under different conditions can be shown by the report on survival of children in falls from heights.[10] Children survived impact velocities of 40 ft/sec on concrete, 51 ft/sec on soil, and 110 ft/sec on water.

The football helmet must combine protection with wearer comfort. It is difficult to fit the variously shaped heads of players with plastic helmets, which have standardized molds of the shell, as special attention is required to fit each helmet individually so that protection is provided to all areas of the head.[1] The helmet shell is selected according to the athlete's head size. The helmet should be snug enough so that it cannot be rotated on the head more than a half inch in either direction. Cheek pads should be fitted to the helmet to occupy the one-quarter- to one-half-inch gap over the cheek on either side. Improving helmet fit on the crown of the head can be accomplished by adjusting the suspension system and adding or removing padding or foam until the front edge of the helmet rides three-quarters of an inch above the eyebrow. The posterior edge of the helmet must provide a three-quarter-inch clearance from the back of the head to allow padding to be added. In addition, the helmet must provide ventilation, especially during hot, humid weather, and even though it is secured to the head throughout all impacts, it must be able to be removed and replaced without a great deal of difficulty. The helmet must be worn by all participants in the game, necessitating that it be reasonable in cost and require low maintenance, either during the season or when stored between seasons. In addition, it must be able to be sanitized and reconditioned when indicated.

The type of helmet selected depends upon the player who will be wearing it. The grade school player, as well as some high school players, does not require the same amount of protection as older, larger athletes because the momentum generated by younger players is far less than that produced by the heavier and faster college and professional athletes. Since increased helmet protection adds weight and bulk, muscle fatigue can result when such a helmet is worn by a younger player with an underdeveloped neck. Other conditions in helmet selection include the shape of the player's head, his position on the team, his aggressiveness, and player preference.

The suspension helmet combines lightness, good ventilation, and easy maintenance but is not always the most comfortable helmet. The padded-suspension helmet is more comfortable but it weighs more. The air helmet is a padded helmet that has inflatable air cells that are inflated after the helmet is on the player's head in order to improve the fit and possibly absorb low-intensity blows. The water helmet has compartments for liquid and is designed to afford greater protection from high-intensity blows. It is heavier than the other helmets and is intended only for the well-conditioned, more experienced athlete.

ADDITIONS TO THE HELMET

Chinstraps

Additions to the helmet shell are necessary for further protection. The chinstrap holds the helmet on the player's head throughout the football play and during all intensities of impact. The concept that the chinstrap should release at certain levels of blows in order to protect the neck is untenable,[9] for, although this line of thinking may work well for ski bindings, in football there is too great a danger of the helmet being lost at a time when the unprotected head would be exposed to multiple blows, and injuries to the head have occurred in such instances when the helmet was accidentally lost during a play. A four-point attachment of the chinstrap to the helmet has been suggested in order to avoid the rocking of the helmet on the head during impact. However, while the helmet must fit securely, some rocking motion of the helmet on impact is desirable in order to provide some "give" to absorb the blow. A chinstrap that prevents such helmet give would increase the chance of injury. The four-point chinstrap, by holding the helmet firmly in place, would prevent nose and neck injuries caused by the sharp frontal and back ridges of the helmet, but padding these areas would accomplish the same objectives while still permitting some desired rocking of the helmet. Regardless of the attachments used, all chinstraps must fit the chin snugly.

Face Mask

The face mask is added to the helmet to protect the face and teeth of the athlete. One of the earliest face masks was made by a blacksmith in 1934, which consisted of a steel crossbar that was laced to the helmet on either side of the face with a center steel bar welded to the center of the crossbar and laced to the helmet at the forehead. This early edition was used because a particular player had recently had his nose operated on and required additional protection. To avoid injury to an opponent from his projecting steel mask, adhesive tape was wrapped around the bar of the mask. This effective, though primitive, device was subsequently replaced by a steel guard encased in rubber. Extending from the crossbar was a semilunar projection intended to protect the teeth. During one particular impact, however, the helmet rocked forward as a result of a blow to the face mask and the extension designed to protect the teeth was responsible for the loss of two front teeth in the player's lower jaw (Fig. 2-7). The face mask, therefore, must project just far enough from the face to avoid this danger, bearing in mind that too great a projection of the mask can be more hazardous than too little, since an increase in the length of the lever arm greatly magnifies the twisting force applied to the neck, as can happen when the face mask is struck or grasped by an opponent. This fact is demonstrated by the example of a nut that can be more easily loosened from its bolt when the handle of an applied wrench is lengthened. Far less force is needed to develop torque when the lever arm is lengthened. At the same time, the face mask must not be securely bolted to the helmet (Fig. 2-8). Rather, it should be attached by plastic loops that can be cut free in order to administer cardiopulmonary resuscitation should the need arise. Unless the face mask can be removed in such an emergency, lifesaving measures cannot be started, as the helmet itself would be very difficult to remove and such removal could very well increase existing injuries.

The face mask does play a significant role in player protection because it prevents facial injuries and a player is not as likely to hit with the crown of the helmet as he would if he had no face mask and had to protect his face. Moreover, players today would be very reluctant to play without the mask. Although the face mask has been criticized for reducing vision, experienced players have not found this to be true. Wearing a face mask for the first time is analagous to wearing eyeglasses for the first time. Initially, the individual is greatly disturbed by the way the glasses interfere with his vision. After getting used to them, however, he is not even aware that he has them on; so it is with the properly fitted face mask.

Everyone concerned with football is interested in the safety of the game and many improvements have been proposed. It seems, however, that most of these changes trade one type of injury potential for another. In order to prevent injury caused by the hard shell of the helmet of one player striking an opponent, it was suggested that the outer surface of the headgear should be covered with padding. Implementing this suggestion resulted in the thickness of padding added to the helmet, extending about two inches on either side of the center of the helmet and reaching from the free edge of the shell in front to the back (Fig. 2-9). This additional padding increased the

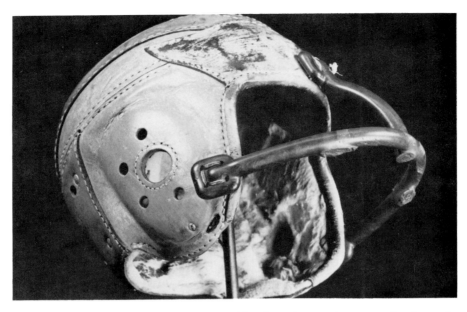

Figure 2-7. On this leather helmet, it is noticeable where the metal protector for the teeth was removed.

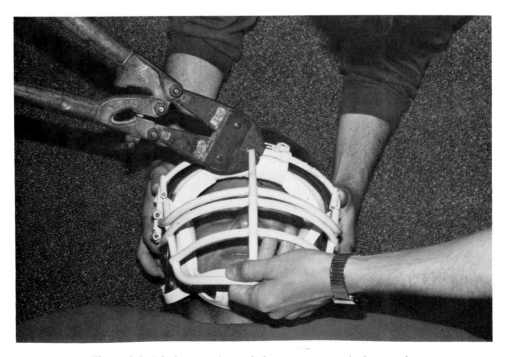

Figure 2-8. A bolt cutter is needed to remove certain face masks.

cost of the helmet and added weight and bulk. Since most blows to the helmet are of a glancing type, a smooth exterior helmet shell causes these blows to slip by without engaging the helmet. The addition of padding would tend to cause the blow to stick, resulting in the forceable twisting of the head, with subsequent head and neck injury. If the athlete is coached against striking with the top of the helmet, what is the rationale for this additional padding?

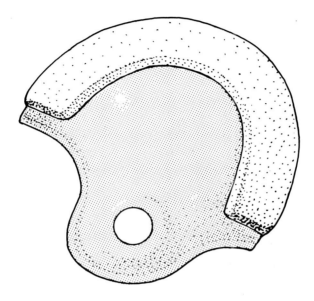

Figure 2-9. Padding may be added to the outside surface of a plastic helmet shell.

Mouth bite is another piece of equipment that should be mandatory in every program. This not only protects the teeth but is instrumental in avoiding cerebral concussions.

Shoulder pad selection is determined by the position played. In general, the inner edge of the shoulder pad should be one-half inch from the neck. The clavicle and the deltoid regions must be protected with additional padding that can be fastened to the shoulder to avoid dislodgement.

Any of the previously described pieces of equipment may be damaged with use, and each piece must be regularly inspected to make sure that all parts are undamaged and still fit properly. Equipment check is the responsibility of each athlete.

SUMMARY

The football helmet has undergone many changes to conform to the demand placed on it by the changing game. Many refinements have been proposed and some of these have been incorporated into the modern helmet, only to find that most of these changes trade one type of injury potential for another. The two protective mechanisms incorporated into a helmet are its ability to spread the force of impact over a greater area of the helmet and to increase the time during which this force is dissipated. The modern plastic helmet utilizes these mechanisms and its capabilities have been clearly demonstrated in very rigid laboratory testing. Far more energy is encountered on the football field than is used to test helmets in the laboratory, but the conditions of the impact are vastly different. The athlete must realize that his own response provides his greatest source of protection. When self-protection gives way to reckless play, the risk of injury is very great. The football helmet cannot provide total protection regardless of its energy-absorbing ability. There is still much room for helmet improvement, but testing must be conducted under more realistic conditions.

REFERENCES

1. Blasco, E. A.: A fit in time saves. *Selling Sporting Goods,* Sept.:95, 1978.
2. Blyth, C. S., and Arnold, D.: Forty-seventh Annual Survey of Football Fatalities, 1931–1978. Copyright 1977 by American Football Coaches Assn., The National Collegiate Athletic Association, and the National Federation of State High School Associations.
3. Gadd, C. W.: Use of a weighted impulse criterion for estimating injury hazard. *Proceedings of the 10th Stapp Car Crash Conference.* Warrendale, PA: Society of Automotive Engineers, Inc., New York, 1966, p. 164.
4. Gurdjian, E. S., Roberts, V. L., and Thomas, L. M.: Tolerance curves of acceleration and intracranial pressure and protective index in experimental head injury. *J Trauma,* 6:600, 1966.
5. Henderson, C. M.: Protective head covering in contact sports. *J National Trainers Assn,* Winter:160, 1971.
6. Hodgson, V. R.: National Operating Committee on Standards for Athletic Equipment: football certification program. *Med Sci Sports,* 7:225, 1975.
7. Reid, S. E., and Reid, S. E., Jr.: Advances in sports medicine. Prevention of head and neck injuries in football. In *Surgery Annual.* New York, Appleton, 1981, Vol. 13, p. 251.
8. Rushmer, R. F., Green, E. L., and Kingsley, H. D.: Internal injuries produced by abrupt deceleration of experimental animals. *J Aviation Med,* Dec. 511, 1946.
9. Schneider, R. C., Reifel, E., Crisler, H. O., and Oosterbann, B. G.: Serious and fatal football injuries involving the head and spinal cord. *JAMA, 177*:362, 1961.
10. Snyder, R. G.: *Impact Injury Tolerance of Infants and Children in Free-fall.* Ann Arbor, Highway Safety Research Institute, University of Michigan, 1970.
11. Snively, G. G., and Chichester, C. O.: Impact survival levels of head acceleration in man. *Aerospace Med, 32*:316, 1961.

Chapter 3

RADIO-TELEMETRY STUDIES OF
HEAD IMPACTS ON THE FOOTBALL FIELD

This chapter has been included in order to describe our experiences in pioneering the recording of the intensity and duration of impacts encountered by a football player during regulation football games. Radio-telemetry was our measuring tool for this study, and it was the first time that telemetry had ever been used in such a vigorous environment. Our study is but a first step in obtaining vital information concerning the tolerance of the living human brain to impact; it is our hope that this information will be useful to others who may be interested in continuing this work, utilizing more sophisticated, miniaturized electronic equipment.

The football field presented an excellent opportunity to measure head impacts on living human beings since in few other situations do individuals willingly submit their heads to such frequent and intense impacts. Our initial problem was finding a means of measuring these impacts during the regularly scheduled games of the Northwestern University Varsity Football Team without encumbering any player's action on the field. This problem was solved by employing the concept of radio-telemetry, which was introduced into the project by the Bio-Medical Engineering Department of the Technological Institute of Northwestern University.

Telemetry means *measured at a distance* and it involves the measurement of some quantity, converting that quantity into an equivalent electrical signal, transmitting the signal to its destination, and then converting the signal into usable form for measurement. The components of our system included transducers that measured the impact encountered by a player, electrodes that recorded the electroencephalogram, signal conditioners, an adder mechanism, a power source, and a transmitter. These components were all carried by one instrumented player. The receiving station in the press box contained the receiver antenna and an FM receiver, an audio recorder for data and spoken comment, a video recorder and camera, a discriminator, and a monitor.[2]

Our original system, which was contained within the football helmet, was designed by the electronic engineers at Northwestern University (Fig. 3-1). A regulation helmet was used throughout the study, and no attempt was ever made to evaluate the efficiency of this helmet. Furthermore, because all impacts were measured at the head of the instrumented player, the amount of a blow absorbed by the helmet was not calculated. Originally, the helmet worn was of the suspension type, consisting of a series of strapped webbings that securely suspended the head within the helmet shell. A space between the head and the shell allowed for head movement as the suspension system stretched to absorb the shock of a blow. This space was adjusted to accommodate the microelectronics of our telemetry system. Engineers at the Technological Institute initially "breadboarded" the system, but it eventually became necessary to have the system built commercially. Manufacturing of electronic equipment that would have an extremely limited market discouraged most firms from accepting the job, but the Government Electronics Division of the Admiral Corporation finally agreed to build the system (Fig. 3-2). A triaxial accelerometer, built by the National Aeronautics and Space Administration (NASA), was acquired to measure accelerations in three mutually perpendicular planes and was secured to the helmet shell with screws. The seed money for this project was provided by the Evanston Hospital and the Northwestern University Medical School. The specifications for the components of the telemetry system and their performance characteristics have been given in tabular form (Tables 3-I, 3-II, 3-III, & 3-IV). A glossary of terms may be found in the Appendix.

As we anticipated, considerable problems were encountered in the fabrication of the system, and the original trial had to be delayed until after the termination of the Northwestern University 1961 football season. The system was tested for the first time in January 1962 during the Pro-Bowl game in the Los Angeles Coliseum, with the helmet being worn by the Detroit Lions' great linebacker, Joe Schmidt. Difficulties arose in signal transmission and we documented these problems for solution later. For example, the transmission of the signal was "line of sight" and we were concerned that the signal might not be captured from the bottom of a pile of players. We felt that it might become necessary to bury wires along the five-yard markers in order to recover the signal. Another problem involved interference from police car radios, citizen band sets, and movie cameras. In addition, we found that when the instrumented player was in a remote corner of the field or had his head in certain orientations with respect to the receiver antenna, the signal was lost. This preliminary test run did, however, establish the feasibility of recording impact data during a football game, and preparations were made to devise more powerful telemetry equipment that could transmit a signal to the press box located 50 to 150 yards away (Fig. 3-3).

In order to form some basis for comparison of our data with statistics obtained by others, it was decided to take the same measurements as those

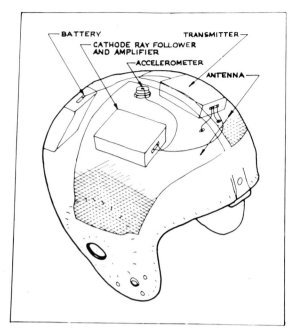

Figure 3-1. A sketch of a helmet with a contained telemetry system.

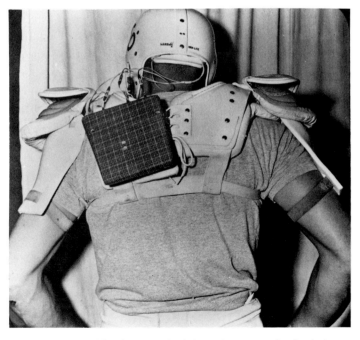

Figure 3-2. Shown here are cables from a triaxial accelerometer in the helmet to the power station on the shoulder pad.

Table 3-I
SPECIFICATIONS OF SENSORS

1. LINEAR ACCELEROMETERS (4)
   Endevco Model 2264 AMI
   Piezoresistive, half-bridge configuration
   Resonance frequency: 80,000 cycles per second
   Not frequency dependent to 36 kilohertz (kilocycles)
   Flat frequency out to two kilohertz (minimum) with no cut-off
   Instrument capacity ± 4500 G's
   Temperature dependence: 3%
   When 330 millivolts used, it has a sensitivity of 310 G/mv according to specification
   Sensitivity range to 740 G
   Frequency range of impacts: 300–800 CPS
   Weight: one gram
   Dimensions: 1.0 cm × 1.0 cm × 0.5 cm
2. FORCE TRANSDUCERS (2)
   Entran load cell
   ELF: 6 – 100 – 250 w
   Range: 250 lbs
   Exitation: 12 volts
   Output: 0.–65 mv/lb
   Input impedance: 4319 ohms
   Output impedance: 796 ohms
   Weight: 14 gms
   Dimensions: 2.5 cm diameter × 0.4 cm
3. EEG ELECTRODES (5)

Table 3-II
TRANSMITTER PACKAGE

1. TRANSMITTER
   Weight: 92 gms
   Dimensions: 6.7 cm × 4.5 cm × 1.7 cm
   Transmitter:
     Carrier power: 90 milliwatts
     Frequency modulated (FM)
     Operating frequency: 236 megahertz
   Amplifiers: 2
   Voltage-controlled oscillators (VCO): 2
2. ANTENNA
   Battery: 9 volts transistor connected to transmitter by a 3-inch wire
   Weight: 42 gms
3. POD
   Compartment on back of helmet
   Slots for insertion of transmitter
   Weight: 163 gms
   Dimensions: 10 cm × 7 cm × 2.8 cm

Table 3-III
ADDITIONAL EQUIPMENT

1. POWER PACK
    Weight: 461 gms
    Dimensions: 13.7 cm × 8.3 cm × 2.5 cm
        Aluminum case
        VCO: 6 accepts only 1 mv full-scale input
        Amplifiers: 6
        Power: Two 10-volt batteries
        Excitation voltage: 0.33
        Adder network
2. PRESS BOX EQUIPMENT
    Receiver: Signatron Engineering: 4200 FM
    Tape recorder: AKAI Cross Field 330 audio; upper limit of frequency response is 3 db roll-off at 22.5
        kilohertz
    Discriminator: Defense Electronics Industries model SCO 11; output adjusted for sensitivity of 0.0088
        volts/g
    Oscilloscope: HP 140 A Bandwidth, 20 megahertz
    Video system: Sony
    Outside antenna
3. LABORATORY EQUIPMENT
    Digital computer
    Sony Videocorder CV-2200
    Sony TV monitor CVM-180µ
    Visacorder: Siemens, six-channel inkjet, 3 db roll-off at 580 hertz

Table 3-IV
SUBCARRIER FREQUENCIES USED IN THIS STUDY

Channel No.	Center Frequency (CPS)	Bandwidth (CPS)	Frequency Response (CPS)	Data Channel
6	1700	± 128	25	E.E.G. − right
7	2300	± 173	35	E.E.G. − left
8	3000	± 225	45	Rotation − left
9	3900	± 293	59	Acceleration − back
10	5400	± 405	81	Acceleration − side
11	7350	± 551	110	Force − back
12	10500	± 788	160	Force − side
13	14500	±1088	220	Rotation − right

Inter-range instrumentation group (IRIG) of the U.S. Department of Defense subcarrier standards.[1]

used by earlier investigators and those presently used in the testing of helmets. The magnitude and duration of accelerations encountered by the head of the player were, therefore, recorded. The additional requirements for power made it necessary to enlarge the system to such a degree that the electronics could not be housed in the very limited space between the head of the player and the shell of the helmet. Consequently, a small compart-

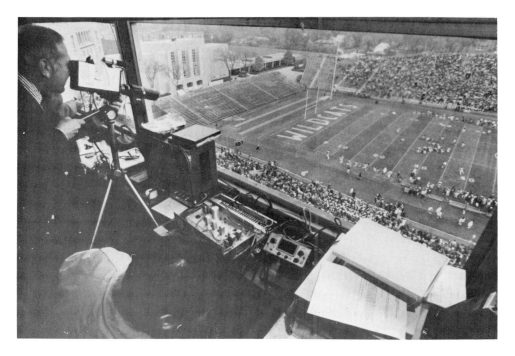

Figure 3-3. The receiving station in the press box and the video camera.

ment or "pod" was attached to the back of the helmet to house the transmitter (Fig. 3-4) and power pack for the additional electronic equipment that was added to the shoulder pad (Fig. 3-5). An umbilical cord connected the electronics of the shoulder pad with the remaining equipment contained in the helmet. Since football is a fall sport, the project was a seasonal study and nine seasons were devoted to develop the telemetry system into its final form, which eventually had the capability of transmitting eight data channels, including six dynamic parameters and one channel of electroencephalography (EEG), from each hemisphere of the brain to monitor the effects of impacts (Fig. 3-6). These eight data channels were recorded on electromagnetic tape and were synchronized with the video action of the player using a telephoto lens.

Problems continued to arise throughout this pioneering study. Since only one player was instrumented, player selection was of paramount importance. Obviously, the player subjected to the largest number of head impacts of the greatest intensity would have been the ideal choice; however, it was not possible to predict who that player might be. We learned that during 50

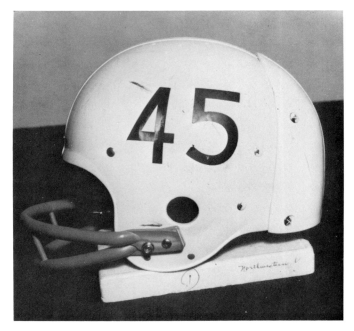

Figure 3-4. Pod at the back of the helmet to house the transmitter.

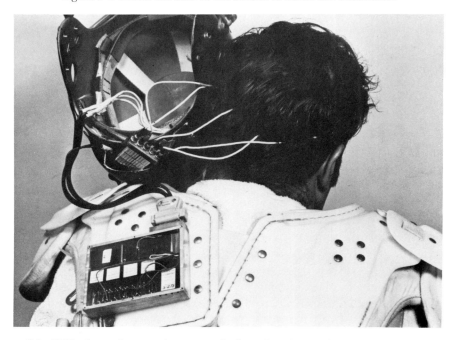

Figure 3-5. EEG electrodes are shown attached to the player's head, which attach to the transmitter partially inserted in the pod.

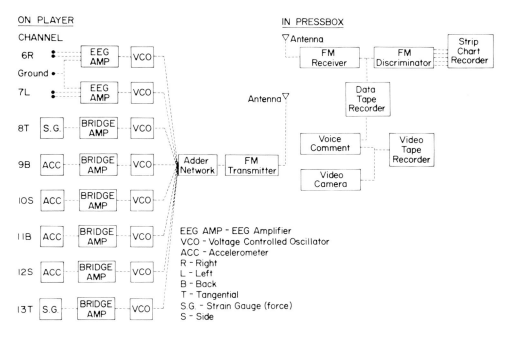

ON PLAYER

CHANNEL

IN PRESSBOX

EEG AMP – EEG Amplifier
VCO – Voltage Controlled Oscillator
ACC – Accelerometer
R – Right
L – Left
B – Back
T – Tangential
S.G. – Strain Gauge (force)
S – Side

Figure 3-6. Diagram of an eight-channel telemetry system and the receiving station in the press box.

percent of all plays a player receives little or no contact, that a player in a certain position on the kicking squad might receive only one high-intensity blow during an entire game, or that the instrumented player might be injured early in the game and would be unable to participate for the balance of the game. As a result, players in several positions were serially instrumented, with the eventual conclusion that the middle linebacker was involved in the most plays and received the greatest percentage of blows. This player, then, became the instrumented player for the duration of the study.

Another problem concerned the time involved to instrument the athlete, which was approximately twenty minutes, and this annoyed the player because it took away from his mental preparation for the game. Early in the study, one player complained to Coach Ara Parseghian that the equipment was a "psychological burden." At this point it would have been easy for Coach Parseghian to have simply told the player to remove the equipment and the study would thus have been terminated. Instead, Coach Parseghian talked to the boy, pointing out that as soon as the game started, he would not even be aware of the fact that he was instrumented. A few years later another player asked Coach Alex Agase if he could remove the equipment, and Coach Agase said he would have to talk to us about the matter. Coach Agase made the suggestion to us that another, less experienced player be instrumented. We explained the importance of instrumenting this particular player and the coach then said he would go back to the boy and talk to him. This resulted in the player agreeing to be instrumented and the study continued.

During out-of-town games, permission from the opposing team was required to instrument the player. These arrangements were always worked out in advance, since a special room near the team locker room was needed to outfit the player and a radio booth in the press box had to be set aside for the receiving equipment. In addition, a letter from Mr. Bill Reed, Commissioner of the Big Ten, was shown to the game officials who routinely came into the locker room to inspect the equipment of all of the players. They were always satisfied that the electronic gear was acceptable. During a game with UCLA, however, the instrumented player proved to be too much for the opposing team. He made tackles behind the line of scrimmage and intercepted passes in the secondary. Northwestern was winning the game when, suddenly, the game was stopped. The instrumented player was brought to our bench by an official, who said the opposing coach believed this player was receiving signals from our coach in the press box. The electronic helmet had to be removed and valuable data was lost.

Problems with the equipment were frequent. On several occasions the umbilical cord running down the back of the player's neck was grasped by an opponent and pulled away from the system, terminating the study for that day. On cold days we had to contend with battery failure, and batteries had to be replaced during the half-time intermissions. Variations in temperature during the season also changed the sensitivity of the transducers and the damping requirement for specific temperature compensation and required adjustments. In addition, electric heating pads were needed for the discriminator in the press box. We were alerted to these problems via an intercom from the press box, and most small problems were corrected while the player was sitting on the bench.

The triaxial accelerometer was originally screwed to the shell of the helmet in our system, but it was soon discovered that the recorded data included the ringing of the plastic shell on impact, and location of the transducer at this site was discontinued. Since no other similar transducer was available that could be safely placed on the surface of the head of the instrumented player, we elected to use linear accelerometers, placing them in orthogonal positions at the back of the head of the player and at a 90 degree angle to this on the right side of the head (Fig. 3-7). These positions were selected over the superior/inferior plane because earlier stages of the study had revealed that less than 5 percent of all impacts were registered on the top of the head, whereas most impacts occurred at the right and left frontal areas of the helmet. During the course of the study, the helmet worn by the player was changed from a suspension type to a padded version. The linear accelerometers were securely fixed to the outside surface of the snugly fitted hatband of the suspension system and, later, to the padding found in the same location. Eastman 910 adhesive cement was used to fix these transducers. One accelerometer measured head acceleration in the front/back plane and a second measured head accelerations in the right/left plane. Small-size angular accelerometers were not available, so we placed a linear accelerometer on each side of the head, aligning its axis of sensitivity in a tangential direction in order to compute angular acceleration. The four linear accelerometers were lightweight and contained in a hermetically sealed case — factors that favorably influenced electronic stability and player acceptance. Finally, a force transducer was added in juxtaposition to each of the orthogonally located linear accelerometers.

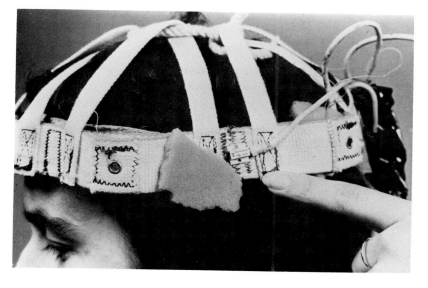

Figure 3-7. The location of the transducer on the suspension system of the helmet is shown.

Two pairs of electrodes, one on each side of the head at the parietal and occipital areas, recorded the electroencephalogram (EEG) (Fig. 3-8). These electrode placements followed the 10–20 system of international electrode placement. A fifth electrode, fixed at the bony prominence at the back of the skull, served as a ground wire. These areas were selected because they were free of underlying muscle that could interfere with the EEG signal and because of the capability of detecting brain effects of impact from slow wave variations of the EEG in these regions. Attachment of the EEG electrodes presented problems. The National Aeronautics and Space Administration (NASA) suggested that we use stick-on electrodes, but this proved unsuccessful. Spring pressure electrodes fixed to the helmet created movement artifacts.[3] It eventually became necessary for us to shave small areas of the scalp in order to attach the electrodes on a player with a crewcut hair style, but we were able to part the hair to get down to the scalp on the player with longer hair and the electrodes were finally firmly secured with multiple applications of preset collodion, each application dried with an airjet. This method proved successful, even during games played in high heat and humidity. Artifacts in the EEG signal due to lead sway were avoided through the application of collodion, not only to the electrodes but to about one inch on the leads from each electrode and by eliminating slack in these leads to the transmitter. These taut leads created a problem in themselves, however, since the player could not remove his helmet until the leads were disconnected from the transmitter. On extremely hot days the discomfort for the instrumented player was significant.

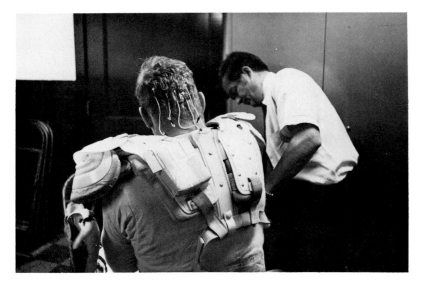

Figure 3-8. EEG electrodes are fixed to the player's scalp with collodion.

The transmitter unit was housed in a special pod fixed to the back of the helmet. Within this pod were slots to secure the transmitter into position. The power supply and additional electronic equipment were housed in an aluminum container that was bolted to the shoulder pad and connected to the rest of the telemetry system in the helmet by a multifunction umbilical cord (Fig. 3-9). The transmitter antenna posed new problems for us, and many types of antennae were tried in various locations. We experimented with flat ribbon foil affixed to the inner surface of the shell of the helmet at the hatband location, incorporating a chinbar heliwhip into the facebar, but these overloaded the transmitter and created noise artifacts. Finally, a simple insulated wire about three inches long was connected to the antenna pole of the transmitter, producing very satisfactory results. Eventually we discovered that a nine-volt battery connected to this three-inch wire produced a far better signal (Fig. 3-10).

All of the components of the telemetry system had to be compatible, and they were adapted for use according to the particular specifications of each. The piezoresistive, half-bridge accelerometer was directly coupled to the VCO, resulting in less sensitivity and noise. The VCO accepted only one millivolt, full-scale input, so extreme sensitivity was not necessary. The half-bridge configuration allowed measurement of comparatively long-term, steady state accelerations, and the resistive-type transducer permitted its placement in the helmet about twelve inches away from the rest of the circuit, located on the shoulder pad, without the interference in the connecting wires associated with a capacitive type of transducer.

Transducer placement was the critical part of our system, since any motion that occurred between the head and the accelerometer could yield incorrect data. Location of the transducers on the helmet shell or any other plastic material of high-frequency response could cause ringing. An attempt was made to place the transducer on an upper molar tooth with the wires protected by the mouthbite, but this location did not receive player acceptance. Accelerometers attached firmly to the outside surface of a snugly fitting headband of the suspension system or to the padding in the helmet would accurately measure head accelerations, although these locations could cause some time lag and would probably damp out the high-frequency response of the skull. When static tests using wooden head models indicated that the acceleration of the headband followed the head model to about ±5 percent, these locations were selected.

The linear accelerometer was also sensitive to the orientation of acceleration and had to be mounted so that most of the head accelerations were in its perpendicular axis. Placement of the accelerometers in mutually perpendicular planes permitted calculation of the vector quantity ($\overline{V}$) from accelerations recorded on each accelerometer on the front (F) and side (S) of the head by the formula $\overline{V} = \sqrt{(F^2 + S^2)}$. When a linear accelerometer was placed on each side of the head, with its axis of sensitivity being aligned tangentially to the rotation of the head and with one transducer recording clockwise rota-

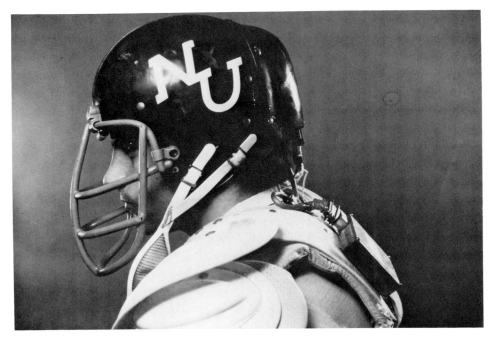

Figure 3-9. A view of the instrumented player before donning his jersey. Courtesy of Appleton-Century-Crofts.

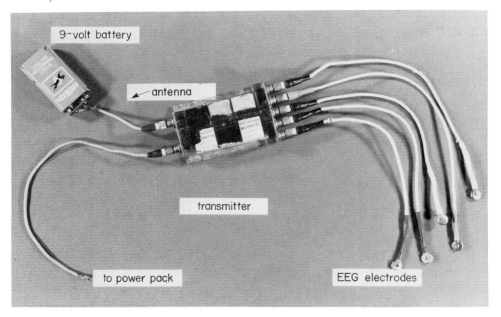

Figure 3-10. Shown here is a transmitter with a three-inch wire and a nine-volt battery attached to the antenna pole.

tion and the other counterclockwise rotation, rotation could be distinguished from translational motion. Angular acceleration in radians per second squared is equal to tangential accelerations in G's over radius of the head in inches or $a = a_t/r$.

The dynamic parameters of accelerations and force are high-frequency responses and required a display vehicle such as an oscilloscope with a 20 megahertz frequency response. Since the composite signal was not a high-frequency response, it could be recorded on an ordinary tape recorder with a 22.5 kilohertz frequency. The half-bridge configuration of the accelerometer and steady state acceleration allowed the system to be calibrated in a small centrifuge. The acceleration (G) in gravitational units is given by the formula: $G = 2.84 \times 10^{-5} rn^2$, where r is equal to the distance in inches from the axis of rotation and n is equal to the revolutions per minute. The uncertainty of the system was governed by the noise level of electronics involved, typically 0.03 volts peak to peak. The error in the accelerometer output, ±7 percent in the worst case, was caused by combination of transducer drift and uncertainties in measuring the values for r and n.

The course of the data signals through the system progressed as follows:

1. Continuous EEG signals were recorded during the time a player was in the game. Because of the difference in the electrical potential between two selected sites on each side of the brain, current flowed between them. This current was then picked up by the EEG electrodes and was conditioned and converted from an AM to an FM signal by its voltage-controlled oscillator (VCO).

2. Acceleration caused a change in resistance in one arm of the Wheatstone bridge in the accelerometer, changing the voltage output of the bridge circuit in a manner proportional to the acceleration.

3. A load cell recorded force in pounds. Pressures were changed to voltage in a manner similar to that of the accelerometer.

4. Bridge output was amplified and directly coupled to a voltage-controlled oscillator (VCO) in the backpack to change voltage output into frequency change. The VCO for each channel was centered on a different subcarrier frequency, and the voltage fed into the VCO was translated into variations in the subcarrier frequency in a linear and reproducible manner.

5. The output of each VCO was multiplexed in an adder network into a single composite signal in such a way that interaction and cross talk between them did not occur. The composite signal modulated the main carrier transmitter, operating at a frequency of 236 megahertz.

6. The receiver in the press box, tuned to 236 megahertz, brought in

the signal and fed this composite signal directly into a tape recorder, as well as into a discriminator which filtered out each different subcarrier frequency and converted these primary signals from frequency changes into the original voltage fluctuations. These voltage outputs were displayed on an oscilloscope as a graph of accelerations or force as functions of time. Later, when further study was done, the taped composite signal could again be fed into the discriminator, and all or any combination of data channels could be displayed on the strip chart or fed into a computer for analysis.

7. The six-channel inkjet recorder proved adequate for the specifications of all our inter-range instrumentation group (IRIG) subcarriers; however, this equipment proved to be too fragile to be moved to out-of-town games, and ink clotting in the jets caused considerable problems. The blue ink used in this recorder produced poor photographic reproductions. A Honeywell recorder had adequate response capability, but the photosensitive paper used in this brand of equipment could be reproduced photographically only with difficulty.

The system was calibrated before each football season. The AC coupled EEG amplifiers were tested by coupling a one millivolt calibration pulse from an electrocardiogram through a 10:1 divider. The calibration used for measuring the acceleration of the entire system was accomplished by the use of a small centrifuge, modified by inserting a small bowl at the center of rotation. The accelerometers were cemented to the bowl, with their axis of sensitivity aligned along a radius of the circle of rotation. The electronics of this system were also secured in the bowl, and the transmitted signals were picked up by telemetry. The system could be rotated briefly for one to two minutes with no ill effects to the electronics, and all four accelerometers could be calibrated at once. Turning the transducers 180 degrees and repeating the measurements gave calibrations in the opposite direction. After calibration by centrifuge, a calibration of the gain in the system was done prior to each game by feeding a one millivolt signal through the system to simulate the accelerometer output.

The force transducers were calibrated by adding known static weights to the transducers and measuring system output. Since force is measured in pounds, the mere addition of weights adequately calibrated the force transducer. A test weight was used before every game to test the system for variations in system gain.

The output from all channels was tested for frequency response by varying the frequency of the test inputs and using an attenuated output from an HP 310 function generator. On all channels the IRIG specifications were satisfied. The frequency response of the inkjet six-channel recorder was tested by matching the data writeout with a picture of the output from an HP 140A oscilloscope with a bandwidth of 20 megahertz. Only if the output matched to ±5 percent was the data accepted.

The upper limit (3 db) of frequency response of the AKAI 330 audio tape recorder was 22.5 kilohertz. Thus, the eight IRIG subcarrier center frequencies that could be recorded were channels 6 to 13 (Table IV). The maximum data cycles per second for these channels ranged from 25 to 220. A study of the effect of the IRIG channel on impact shape was made by allowing a weighted hammer to fall on a given spot on the helmet and comparing the output of the same accelerometer connected to each VCO in turn. There was a 10 percent deviation between each data frequency response and channel bandwidth in both amplitude, 80 G's, and duration, 40 milliseconds, and the wave shapes were very similar for all tests. The tests that were devised to verify our results have, to date, not uncovered any systematic error.

SUMMARY

The concept of using radio-telemetry to measure the intensity and characteristics of blows to the head and neck occurring in football was first employed in a twenty-year seasonal study conducted jointly by the Evanston Hospital and Northwestern University. The football field became our laboratory; the middle linebacker for the Northwestern University Football Team was our test subject. Our goal in this study was to obtain vital, but previously unavailable information regarding the tolerance of the human brain to impact. This textbook details many of our findings, and this chapter describes in depth the telemetry system that we developed, the problems we encountered, and the solutions we devised. Our aim in presenting this information is to encourage other researchers to continue on with this pioneering study, utilizing the more sophisticated electronic equipment that is available today.

APPENDIX

DEFINITIONS OF TERMS USED IN THIS CHAPTER

ADDER MECHANISM: A linear mixing network that combines all the VCO outputs in such a manner that interaction and cross talk between channels do not occur.

CYCLE: A single round trip of an oscillating body.

DECIBEL (DB): Used as a unit for the logarithmic expression of ratios of power, voltage, or current in radio communication.

DISCRIMINATOR: A network used to demodulate the subcarriers to convert the changes of subcarrier frequency to an output voltage that has the same variations used at the transmitting end of the system.

FREQUENCY: The number of oscillations or cycles per unit of time.

MODULATE: Change in frequency of electrical waves by imposing upon them other waves of another, usually lower, frequency. This term has a broader meaning that includes changes in the voltage output of the accelerometer into variations in subcarrier frequency in a linear and reproducible manner.

RESONANCE: The natural frequency of a body in motion. For example, when the accelerations of the shell of the helmet vibrate at a frequency equal to that of the accelerometer, the natural frequency of the accelerometer is reached, resulting in an increased amplitude of response, which causes ringing or re-echoing and produces false results. To avoid resonance frequency, the object measured must have a frequency of less than 20 percent of the resonance of the accelerometer.

SIGNAL CONDITIONER: Equipment used to convert the measured quantity into a form suitable for transmission or to amplify the signal.

REFERENCES

1. Andrews, A.: *ABC's of Telemetry.* Indianapolis, Sams, 1968.
2. Foster, L. E.: *Telemetry Systems.* New York, Wiley, 1965.
3. Westbrook, R. M., and Zaccaro, J. J.: Helmet system broadcasts electroencephalograms of wearer. *NASA Technical Brief* #66-10536, 1966.

Chapter 4

PARAMETERS OF MOTION

This chapter is included to promote insight into the mechanism of head protection and to discuss the parameters of motion that apply to collision between two bodies as they relate to impacts on the football field.

Engineers must know the tolerance of the living human brain to impact in order to improve upon the modern football helmet. This information is not available at the present time because man is unwilling to voluntarily subject his head to potentially lethal blows, especially since it is known that a head injury can occur at a level of intensity far below what is thought to be tolerable. Furthermore, impact data reported from the laboratory has been developed under very specific conditions, and this data proves unreliable under different experimental conditions. For example, Holbourn[4] reported that head injury is proportional to change in velocity when the blow is of short duration, but brain injury is proportional to acceleration with blows of long duration. This analysis is based on the assumption that the brain and its restraints follow the physical laws governing the action of a spring mass system. Recognized authorities state that among the head response indices, only linear acceleration shows significant correlation with concussion,[1] while equally reputable investigators find that there is no correlation between severity of the concussive effect and magnitude of acceleration. Lissner[5] reported that an increase in the time duration of an impact greatly magnifies the intensity of the blow, but Rushmer[7] found that when a change in velocity occurs in a very short time, forces are produced that are beyond comprehension and that more severe injuries are associated with force acting for very brief periods.

Clearly, it is important to determine the parameters of motion that will accurately record brain tolerance under specific conditions and to determine the intensity of blows that occur in situations where head protection is used. The helmet must have shock-absorbing capabilities to match the intensity of the impact in order to give the human brain a smooth ride through a football game. Just as a sports car equipped with shock absorbers designed for a truck would give the driver a very rough ride over an uneven road, a football helmet with shock-absorbing characteristics that are not designed to fit the range of blows encountered on the football field could cause recurrent commotion of cellular structures in the brain of the player.

An impact is a blow resulting from a collision of two bodies. Its intensity is measured by the force that is exerted, and this force is equal to the resistance of an object to being moved and the rapidity of the change in motion. Motion itself is not injurious, and no force is required to keep a body moving if no resistance is encountered. For example, riding along in an automobile causes no unpleasant sensation until there is a change in either the direction or in the speed of the vehicle. Force, expressed in pounds, is measured according to Newton's three laws of motion involving mass, change in velocity, accelerations, and time. The resistance of an object to being moved is dependent upon the weight of the object. Since the weight of the object is a measure of the pull of gravity to earth, its weight will vary with the distance of the object from the center of gravity of the earth. For example, the astronauts on the moon were in a relatively weightless state because the earth's attraction is far less on the moon than on the surface of the earth. To compensate for this difference in the pull of gravity in various locations, mass is used instead of weight as a measure of resistance. The pull of gravity on the surface of the earth varies, but in this discussion it will be considered to be exactly 32 ft/sec^2, or one gravitational unit (G). The impact in a fall is more severe than that experienced as a result of a collision between two bodies, because there is no "give" to the earth and no transference of energy is possible. It has been estimated that twice the amount of energy is required to produce the same concussive effect between two bodies of equal masses as would occur in a fall of one of those bodies to earth.[6]

NEWTON'S FIRST LAW OF MOTION

$$F = \frac{M\Delta V}{t}$$

F = FORCE EXPRESSED IN POUNDS

M = MASS EXPRESSED IN SLUGS

$\quad = \dfrac{W}{G}$

W = WEIGHT IN POUNDS

G = ONE GRAVITATIONAL UNIT

$\quad$ = 32 FT/SEC/SEC (32 FT/SEC^2)

ΔV = CHANGE IN VELOCITY IN ft/SEC

t = TIME IN SECONDS

$$
\boxed{
\begin{array}{l}
\text{NEWTON'S SECOND LAW OF MOTION} \\[4pt]
F = M \times A \\[4pt]
\quad A = \text{ACCELERATION OR} \\
\qquad \text{DECELERATION IN} \\
\qquad \text{FT/SEC}^2 \\[6pt]
\quad M = \dfrac{F}{A}
\end{array}
}
$$

Change in motion is measured by change in velocity or by acceleration or deceleration. Velocity is speed in a given direction, and any change in velocity, either in speed or direction, requires a force to effect this change. A change in velocity is no indication of the involved force unless the time during which this change occurs is given. Change in velocity may occur from a position of rest or from an increase or decrease in an existing state of motion. Acceleration, on the other hand, is a change in velocity per unit of time and is an index of the response of an object to the force applied to it or of the energy dissipation after impact. The relationship between acceleration and change in velocity is derived from Newton's first two laws of motion. For example, a change in velocity from 10 ft/sec to 30 ft/sec equals 20 ft/sec, and if this change occurred in 0.010 sec the acceleration would be 2,000 ft/sec^2. This large number is more conveniently expressed in gravitational units as 62.5 G's.

$$
\boxed{
\begin{array}{c}
F = \dfrac{M\Delta V}{t} = M \times A \\[8pt]
\text{WHEN M IS CONSTANT} \\[6pt]
A = \dfrac{\Delta V}{t}
\end{array}
}
$$

Inertia is the resistance of a mass to being moved, while momentum is a resistance of a moving mass to being stopped. Momentum is a more complete term for an object in motion than is velocity, because momentum includes the measurement of the mass of the object. For example, greater injury could result if a man were struck by a two-ton automobile travelling thirty miles per hour than if he were hit by a bicycle travelling at the same speed. When one body exerts a force on a second body in a collision, the second body simultaneously exerts a force on the first body. These forces are equal in magnitude but are opposite in direction. Either force may be considered the action and the other the reaction. A mutual, simultaneous interaction of forces is implied. In a collision of rigid bodies, very little is known about the events that take place during the actual very brief period of the collision, but much is gained by studying the before and after situations utilizing the principles of conservation of momentum. Momentum is imparted to a body by a constant force acting for a period of time. The longer the time this force acts, the greater is the momentum.

$$MOMENTUM = MV$$
$$CONSERVATION\ OF\ MOMENTUM\ IN\ IMPACT$$
$$MV = MV$$
$$NEWTON'S\ THIRD\ LAW$$
$$ft = \Delta MV$$
$$Ft = IMPULSE\ IN\ POUND\text{-}SECONDS$$
$$\Delta MV = CHANGE\ IN\ MOMENTUM$$

When an object is dropped from a height, the falling time determines the momentum imparted to the mass of the object. A 16-pound weight (0.5 slugs) dropped from a 4-foot height has an impact velocity of 16 ft/sec ($V = \sqrt{2Gh}$) and an average velocity of 8 ft/sec. Therefore, to fall four feet the falling time is 0.5 second, and the greater the height of the drop, the longer the falling time and the greater is the momentum at impact. To stop this falling object, a counterforce is exerted at impact and it is inversely proportional to the stopping time. The longer the stopping time, the less counterforce required at impact. The time, therefore, required to gain momentum must not be mistaken for the stopping time of the momentum. This same principle of physics applies to the batter in baseball. When the batter strikes the ball, he drives it off into the field. The amount of force applied to the ball remains the same, but if the batter follows through on the swing of the bat, he applies this force to the ball for a longer period of time than he would if he stopped his swing when only halfway through. The longer the swing time, the greater is the force, or momentum, imparted to the ball. The counterforce the fielder uses depends on the length of time he takes to stop the ball in the padding of his gloved hand. The padding increases the stopping time to a certain extent, but if the fielder allows his gloved hand to move with the ball, the stopping time is greatly increased and the counterforce is markedly reduced.

In our introductory discussion of head injuries, rotational movements of the head were cited as the main cause of injury. A brief discussion of these units of motion is necessary to understand the mechanism involved. These terms include torque, angular acceleration, angular velocity, and moment of inertia. Rotational changes are measured according to Newton's laws of motion, with rotational analogues substituted for linear parameters. For example, torque or moment of force is substituted for force, and moment of inertia is substituted for mass. Rotational movement occurs around a pivotal point, and the larger the circle of rotation, the smaller is the curvature along the periphery of the circle. The rotational movement is, therefore, directly related to the angle of the circle traversed. It would be inconvenient to refer to degrees of angles in such a discussion and a simpler unit has been developed. The unit is the radian and it is based on the equation for the circumference of a circle. It is the length of the arc along the periphery of a pie-shaped segment of the circle having an angle of 57.3 degrees. Thus, the radian would be of different lengths for different-sized circles, but the rotational movement would be the same. Rotational movements then are recorded not in feet but in radians. For example, linear acceleration is recorded in feet per second squared, but rotational acceleration is recorded in radians per second squared. Rotational accelerations are measured by an angular accelerometer, but tangential accelerations can be converted to angular accelerations.

CIRCUMFERENCE OF A CIRCLE

$2\Pi R$

$\Pi = 3.1416$

R = RADIUS OF CIRCLE

2Π RADIANS = 360°

ONE RADIAN = 57.3°

Θ – ANGLE EXPRESSED IN RADIANS

$\propto$ = ANGULAR ACCELERATIONS IN RADIANS/SEC^2

$$\propto = \frac{\text{TANGENTIAL ACCELERATIONS (G)}}{\text{RADIUS OF CIRCLE IN INCHES}}$$

Newton's laws of motion apply to laboratory testing of helmets. The helmet is fitted to an artificial head form calculated to weigh the equivalent of an amputated human head (11 lbs). Impacts to this weighted helmet are simulated in the laboratory using a simple pendulum or by means of a guided free-fall onto a 300-pound platform. The pendulum consists of a mass (bob) fixed to a wire, which causes the bob to swing along an arc. The force developed in such an apparatus is the restoring force created by displacing the bob from its neutral or perpendicular position. Impacts to the helmet are most often measured by the guided drop method, and this is the method currently used by the National Operating Committee for Standards in Athletic Equipment (NOCSAE).[3] This measurement, however, is not very accurate, since air resistance and the resistance created by the guided drop cannot be calculated. The method of conversion of energy into a force measurement is included in the Appendix to compare these quantities.[2,8] In actual helmet testing, the impact is measured by an accelerometer secured at the center of gravity of the head form. These helmet tests are performed under static conditions so that all the energy in the system is absorbed by the helmet. This, then, is a true test of the helmet material. The fact that the weighted helmet remains the same with all tests, and the fact that the stopping time of the blow remains constant, means that the only variable to be recorded is acceleration.

The original head forms were made of rigid material in order to accurately test the energy-absorbing characteristics of helmets. It was mentioned earlier in the text that a force applied to a body causes a change in the state of its motion, but, in addition, force also causes a distortion from the normal shape of the body. This local deforming motion adds little to the response of the body as a whole and furthermore is a very difficult measurement to make in a dynamic environment. Nevertheless, the local response of material to an applied force will be briefly touched upon here because of its application to the newly devised head form presently used for helmet testing. The ratio of force applied to a body is the stress exerted, and this stress is directly proportional to the distortion or strain. This ratio is constant for a given material, provided its elastic limit is not exceeded. Rigid bodies, such as billiard balls, are almost perfectly elastic, distort with difficulty when they collide, and very little energy is dissipated during the brief contact time. An example of materials that are perfectly inelastic are viscous bodies, since when viscous bodies collide they return to their original shape only after a delayed period of time or they may even stick together and move as a single unit. Energy is absorbed during this prolonged period. The local reaction of living tissue varies between the behavior of elastic and inelastic bodies and is classified as a visco-elastic response. Impacts to the human head normally can cause distortion of the skull and brain without any injurious effects. These response characteristics are incorporated into the present head form used in helmet testing and have resulted in some increase in the stopping time of the momentum of the blow.[3]

Measurements of impacts made in the laboratory under controlled conditions are difficult to interpret, and the difficulty increases when one attempts to measure impacts of collisions in the dynamic environment of a football field. Impacts are unpredictable; they can come from all directions and strike the helmet in a variety of ways. The forces encountered are produced by man (the charging player) and, therefore, are within man's ability to defend. The force is not the simple accelerating force that is encountered in a drop from a height, but it is the *sustaining charge* of the athlete who continues to generate force even during impact. This force is the result of the momentum developed by the charging player and it is opposed by the athlete who has been trained to resist a charge. This increased resistance is equivalent to an increase in mass and is referred to as the effective mass involved in the impact. This increased mass, demonstrated by Newton's second law of motion, decreases acceleration, thereby reducing the injurious effects of the impact. The increased mass also causes an increase in the stopping time of the blow, which is demonstrated by Newton's first law. In a situation such as this, involving a variable mass, Newton's second law cannot be applied except as a measurement of the force at any specific moment. The force of the entire impact can be calculated using Newton's first law. Furthermore, the relation between acceleration and change in velocity does not apply under conditions where a variable mass exists and when Newton's two laws cannot be used interchangeably.

With all these variable parameters of motion, how then can measurements be made in a collision that may involve one athlete in motion while the opposing player is at rest or in situations where both players are in motion? Certainly measurements only of acceleration and/or change in velocity would not give a true picture of the response or of the force of the impact. There is one principle that can be applied to the measurement of variable motion and that is the principle of conservation of momentum, one of the most important principles of mechanics. The change in momentum of one player equals the change in momentum of the opposing player in a collision between two athletes whose masses and changes in velocity vary. The force required to change momentum is a function of time and it is the impulse. This is the impulse-momentum thorem. This equation is applicable here because, since both the mass and change in velocity are variable, even their product would be quite difficult to calculate, but the impulse (the equivalent of change in momentum) can be measured. (Force as the integral of time is represented as the area under the force-time curve.) This value can be readily calculated. The recorded time is the interval during which the momentum is reduced to zero, and this is the stopping time. From the impulse-momentum relationship, it can be seen that force is inversely proportional to time and that an extremely great force would be required to reduce a given momentum to zero within ten milliseconds, which is the typical time recorded for impacts to rigid bodies. However, with the relatively prolonged stopping time of about 300 milliseconds, which has been recorded by telemetry, far less counterforce would be required to change the same momentum to zero. For example, the same counterforce that is required to reduce the given momentum to zero in seven milliseconds could reduce a momentum 40 times this magnitude to zero within 300 milliseconds. This seemingly unbelievable effect of prolonging the stopping time is consistent with the finding that the same helmet that tests to less than 90 foot-pounds of energy under the rigid conditions of the laboratory can be subjected to about 40 times this energy on the football field when a 224-pound athlete traveling 100 yards in 10 seconds delivers 3,150 foot-pounds of energy upon collision with an opponent. It is believed that high impacts can occur on the football field, but fortunately these are rarely encountered because injuries occur so infrequently. A more plausible explanation for the fact that injury is often avoided is that the stopping time of these high-intensity impacts is prolonged far beyond the time measured when inanimate objects collide. The force involved in football is not a *single* high measurement of a quantity that has to be dissipated over a long period of time; it is a variable force that is being generated all during the impact as the athlete *sustains* his drive and meets *sustained* resistance from his opponent.

SUMMARY

This somewhat simplified description of the fundamentals of physics that apply to football field impacts can be summarized to a few brief statements. All motion can be expressed using Newton's three laws, which involve force, mass, change in velocity, acceleration, and time. The fact that a football player increases his resistance to a charging player creates a variable mass that changes the conditions from a rigid environment to a dynamic setting. The point must be emphasized that a single, high one-time force, similar to that of a flying object, is not the force delivered by the sustained charge of a football player. The player strikes with a definite force as his legs continue to churn to develop additional force to overcome the sustained resistance of his opponent.

APPENDIX

Conversion of Energy to Force

Potential energy: $E_p = MGh$
Kinetic energy: $E_k = \frac{1}{2}MV^2$
Change in momentum $= \Delta MV$
Impulse $= Ft$
    $Ft = \Delta MV$
Example: Helmet dropped from height to a platform
    Initial height: $E_p \doteq MGh$, $E_k = 0$
    Impact surface: $E_p = 0$, $E_k = \frac{1}{2}MV^2$
      $MGh = \frac{1}{2}MV^2$
      $2Gh = V^2$
      $\sqrt{2Gh} = V$ = velocity of helmet at impact surface
    $Ft = \Delta MV$
    $F = M\, (\sqrt{[Gh]} - 0)/t$
    $F = M\sqrt{2Gh}/t$
    where t = time to stop helmet at impact

REFERENCES

1. Gold, A. J., Hance, H. E., Kornhauser, M., and Lawton, R. W.: Impact tolerance of restrained mice as a function of velocity change and average acceleration. *Aerospace Med, 33*:204, 1962.
2. Halliday, D., and Resnick, R.: *Fundamentals of Physics.* New York, Wiley, 1974.
3. Hodgson, U. R.: National Operating Committee on Standards for Athletic Equipment: football certification program. *Med Sci Sports, 7*:225, 1975.
4. Holbourn, A. H.: Mechanics of head injuries. *Lancet, 2*:438, 1943.
5. Lissner, H. R., Lebow, M., and Evans, F. G.: Experimental studies on relation between acceleration and intracranial pressure changes in man. *Surg Gynecol Obstet, 111*:329, 1960.
6. Rayne, J. M., and Maslin, K. R.: Factors in the design of protective helmets. *Aerospace Med, 40*:631, 1969.
7. Rushmer, R. F., Green, E. L., and Kingsley, H. D.: Internal injuries produced by abrupt deceleration of experimental animal. *J Aviation Med,* December: 511, 1946.
8. Tipler, P. A.: *Physics.* New York, Worth, 1976.

Chapter 5

ANALYSIS OF TELEMETRY DATA

Our purpose in compiling telemetry data from the football field was to obtain information on the brain's tolerance to impact and to compare this with helmet test data. Once we developed the tools for collecting impact data, we had to determine which parameters of motion needed to be measured to yield this information. Impact acceleration was one of the parameters of motion we measured. When a player is hit, the *magnitude* of the impact, as well as the player's method of response to it, are calculated by measuring the resultant acceleration of the head and neck of the athlete. Impact *duration,* another parameter of motion measured in our study, determines the type of injury sustained. After analyzing data obtained during several football seasons, one important conclusion was evident. Specifically, our studies demonstrated that the accepted limits of brain tolerance determined by in vitro laboratory tests were significantly lower than the limits calculated by means of in vivo studies conducted on the football field.

ACCELERATION–TIME CURVE

Measurement of acceleration and duration was accomplished through the use of accelerometers. These measurements were then recorded in coordinate geometry as X–Y graphs, where the magnitude of acceleration was plotted in G's against the time measured in milliseconds (Fig. 5-1), and change in velocity (the product of the average acceleration and elapsed time) was computed by measuring the area under the curve.

An analysis of the acceleration-time curve made during impact revealed that as long as the points along the curve were above the baseline, acceleration was occurring, with the points moving farther away from the baseline as acceleration increased to its peak. When the acceleration curve flattened out, acceleration had reached a constant value. Once peak acceleration had occurred, acceleration began to decrease until the curve returned to the baseline of the graph, whereupon acceleration ceased, although velocity continued. As the curve extended beneath the baseline, velocity diminished and finally ceased. With regard to injury, impacts of short duration caused structural damage proportional to change in velocity, injuries such as skull fractures, or shearing neck injuries with associated intervertebral joint

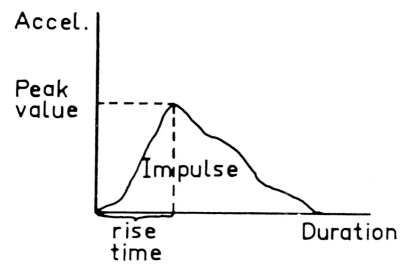

Figure 5-1. Example of an acceleration pulse. Impulse is time integral of acceleration or change in velocity.

dislocation. Impacts of long duration produced brain injuries proportional to acceleration.

The significant features of the acceleration-time curve are: (1) rate of onset; (2) peak or plateau of acceleration; (3) duration of the peak or plateau; (4) duration from onset to the return of the curve to its baseline; and (5) force direction. The rate of onset or rise time of acceleration is represented by the steep climb to a peak acceleration. A sharp rise time to a peak of acceleration is an important cause of skull fracture and may modify the acceleration value at which damage occurs.[16,5] The character of the acceleration-time curve depends upon the duration of acceleration, with many curve variations possible. Acceleration may grow to a point and then immediately return to the baseline, forming a single peak, or multiple peaks can occur during one impact.

The duration of the acceleration-time curve begins when the curve leaves the baseline and continues until it returns to the baseline. Effective acceleration, on the other hand, refers only to the duration of the peak or plateau of the curve; it does not include the rise or return time. Effective acceleration is an average of all accelerations occurring during a single impact. Finally, the initial direction of the takeoff of the curve from the baseline indicates the direction of impact (Fig. 5-2).

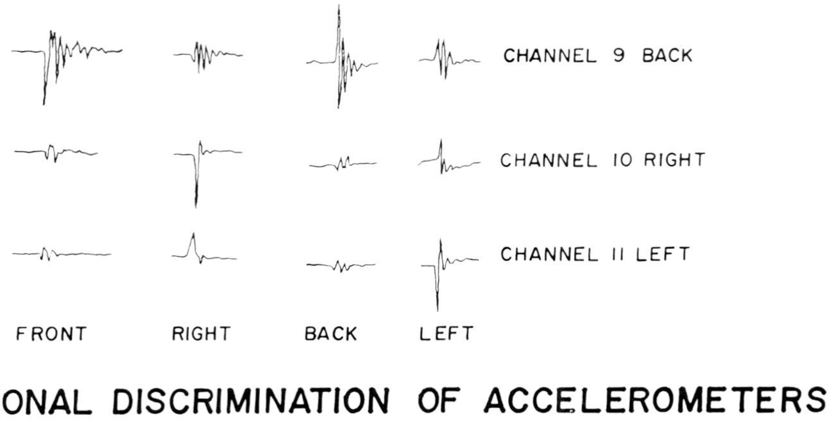

CHANNEL 9 BACK

CHANNEL 10 RIGHT

CHANNEL 11 LEFT

FRONT   RIGHT   BACK   LEFT

DIRECTIONAL DISCRIMINATION OF ACCELEROMETERS

Figure 5-2. This illustration shows the direction of takeoff of waves from the baseline recording of each accelerometer when a blow is struck on the front, back, or sides of the head and locates the point of impingement of a blow on the head.

Instruments for Measurement

In the initial phase of the study, a triaxial accelerometer, fixed to the inner surface of the shell of the helmet, allowed us to record the measured acceleration and the duration of impact (Fig. 5-3). This data has been summarized in Table 5-I and demonstrates peak values ranging from 71 to 5,760 G's, with the highest G values invariably associated with the smallest time interval. Conversely, the greatest pulse duration was always associated with the lowest G values. G values in 87 percent of the recorded impacts registered below 400 G's, with only 8 percent in the 400 to 1,000 range and only 5 percent above 1,000 G's. Impact durations ranged from 1 to 150 milliseconds, with most lasting 2 milliseconds (Table 5-II). In addition, our data revealed that most of the impacts occurred on the sides of the helmet, several occurred on the front, but very few occurred on the top of the helmet. Finally, in 50 percent of the plays the athlete received no contact whatsoever (Table 5-III).

We prepared for our in vivo studies on the football field by conducting laboratory tests to study the damping effect of the helmet. The helmet was mounted on a dummy head, and blows of varying intensity were delivered to various spots on the helmet as the G measurements were recorded. An accelerometer was then moved around on the helmet in ever-enlarging perimeters in order to pinpoint acceleration falloff produced by varying amounts of force delivered at one point on the shell. From these tests, the damping effect of the helmet could be calibrated. This data demonstrated

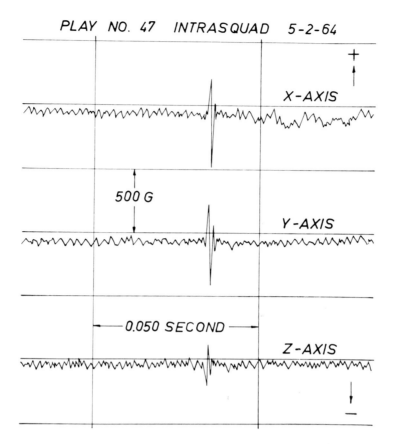

PLAY NO. 47   INTRASQUAD   5-2-64

X-AXIS

500 G

Y-AXIS

0.050 SECOND

Z-AXIS

Figure 5-3. Triaxial accelerometer recording of a blow to the head, which activated its three mutually perpendicular axes.

that the triaxial accelerometer fixed to the shell of the helmet recorded shell vibrations and deformation while failing to record head acceleration with any degree of accuracy.

Proper placement of the accelerometer on the player's head was essential. Any motion at the interface between the accelerometer and the player's head produced noise artifacts that masked impact data. Because, as we mentioned, very few impacts actually occur to the top of the head, we decided to place the linear accelerometers in orthogonal positions only on the front and sides of the outer surface of the snugly fitting headband of the suspension system of the helmet. This permitted us to calculate the vector quantity of the highest peak measured by each accelerometer ($\overline{V} = V[F^2 + S^2]$). It should be noted here that the material in the headband of the suspension system tended to damp rather than resonate the vibrations. Although multiple

Head and Neck Injuries in Sports

Table 5 - I

FREQUENCY AND MAGNITUDE OF ACCELERATIONS TO HELMET

G RANGE	FREQUENCY							
	Northwestern vs Indiana	Northwestern vs Illinois	Northwestern vs Minnesota	Northwestern vs Miami (Ohio)	Northwestern vs Michigan State	Northwestern vs Michigan	Northwestern vs Wisconsin	Northwestern vs Ohio State
0- 100			3					1
100- 200	8	6	23	1	5	21	12	24
200- 300	7	22	14		16	7	12	8
300- 400	5	11	11	2	15		1	5
400- 500	2		1		2	4		1
500- 600	2						1	1
600- 700	1	2	1		1			
700- 800	1	1						
800- 900	1							
900-1000	1	1		1				
1000-2000	1		2					
2000-3000	1	1						
3000-4000	1		1	1		1	1	1
4000-5000								
5000-6000	1							3
TOTAL NUMBER PLAYS	32/97	44/80	56/118	5/33	39/59	33/45	27/54	44/62
PERCENTAGE BLOWS PER GAME PLAYS PARTICIPATED IN	33.0	55.0	47.4	15.3	66.1	73.3	50.0	71.0

Table 5 - II

ACCELERATION DISTRIBUTION OF BLOWS TO FOOTBALL HELMET

G-RANGE	FREQUENCY	DURATION IN MILLISECONDS
0-400	781	1-150
401-1000	61	1-30
OVER 1000	51	1-4

acceleration peaks of varying amplitude occurred during a single impact, we decided to measure only the single highest peak in order to compare our data with that obtained from the in vitro helmet testing. The duration of impact was measured in milliseconds. EEG recordings were added to the system to monitor the effects of brain impacts by recording changes in the basic background rhythm.[12,6] It should be mentioned here that two EEG channels provide insufficient information to pinpoint localized brain damage. These two channels can, however, reveal abnormal patterns and/or disturb-

Table 5 - III

DISTRIBUTION OF BLOWS
RADIO TELEMETRY DATA FROM
NORTHWESTERN — 1963 SEASON

OPPONENT	DATE	FRONT*	BACK*	LEFT SIDE*	RIGHT SIDE*	TOP*
Indiana	9/28	6	0	10	14	2
Illinois	10/5	0	0	30	12	1
Minnesota	10/12	5	1	21	26	3
Miami (Ohio)	10/19	3	0	0	2	0
Michigan State	10/26	1	1	17	20	0
Michigan	11/2	1	1	21	6	3
Wisconsin	11/9	2	0	11	13	1
Ohio State	11/16	2	2	19	18	3
TOTAL BLOWS		20	5	129	111	13

*Front, Back, Left, Right, and Top correspond to core parting line marks on interior of helmet.

ances in other normal brain rhythms. Such information is clinically useful in monitoring these brain disturbances.[2]

On-Field Measurements

With the accelerometers fixed to the suspension system of the helmet, we measured 650 impacts during the 1963, 1964, and 1965 football seasons. These impacts ranged in intensity from 40 G's to 530 G's, with the duration ranging from 20 to 420 milliseconds (Table 5-IV). During the 1970 Northwestern University football season, the instrumented player, a middle linebacker, participated in 418 plays during seven Big Ten Conference games and received a total of 169 measured head impacts (Table 5-V). The peak acceleration of these impacts ranged from 40 G's to 230 G's, with a time duration of 20 milliseconds to 420 milliseconds. These impacts were evenly distributed between the right and left sides of his head, and almost all had an appreciable frontal component.

A scattergram of the 15 highest-intensity impacts is presented in Figure 5-4. Five of these impacts ranged from 188 to 230 G's, with a duration of 310 to 370 milliseconds. One of these resulted in a concussion, while the remaining four caused no abnormalities, either clinically or in the EEG recording. Telemetry of the concussion-producing play (Fig. 5-5) demonstrated an acceleration peak of 188 G's lasting 310 milliseconds involving the left frontal area of the head. Electroencephalographic tracing immediately following injury was compared with the tracing taken at rest after an earlier play and a noticeable difference in the tracing of the right side of the brain could be seen (Fig. 5-6). Specifically, a definite flattening of the wave on the right side of the brain opposite the side of the head that received the blow was demonstrated. In the EEG taken three days later, bilateral spikes were

Table 5 – IV

DISTRIBUTION OF 650 MEASURED IMPACTS
VECTOR PEAK IN G's

DURATION-MILLISECONDS	0-50	51-100	101-150	151-200	201-250	251-300	301-350	351-400	401-450	451-500	501-550
0-50	17	16	15	10	15	8	5	6	5	0	0
51-100	13	58	80	76	37	18	17	21	14	9	3
101-150	0	3	6	11	11	2	4	11	3	0	0
151-200	0	6	35	26	13	6	5	4	1	1	0
201-250	0	0	2	4	4	1	4	1	0	0	0
251-300	1	0	4	11	6	3	0	1	1	2	0
301-350	0	0	0	1	2	1	0	1	0	0	0
351-400	0	1	1	4	1	1	1	0	0	0	0

Table 5-V
DISTRIBUTION OF 169 MEASURED IMPACTS TO ONE PLAYER

Duration (msecs)	Vector peak in G's				
	0–50	51–100	101–150	151–200	201–230
0–100	5	30	32	22	4
101–200	0	6	31	16	3
201–300	0	0	4	9	1
301–400	0	0	0	4	1
401–420	0	0	1	0	0

seen in both posterior temporal areas, with a mild slow wave disorder seen on the frontal occipital, and left temporal areas (Fig. 5-7).

Our telemetry studies of head impacts occurring on the football field presented us with seemingly inconsistent information. One instrumented player received four impacts of at least equal intensity and suffered no injury as a result of these impacts. A fifth impact, however, which was of intensity comparable to the previous four, caused concussion. In order to reconcile this seeming contradiction, factors other than impact intensity needed to be analyzed to determine which variables caused the concussion. The additional factors we analyzed were: (1) variable mass, (2) rotational acceleration, (3) cumulative effect of repeated blows, (4) cervical cord stretching, and (5) erroneous data.

The effective mass is the measure of varying resistance offered by the player. Although mass was not measured in the concussion-producing play, the stop-action film (Fig. 5-8) showed the player spinning out of the block of two opponents and driving his head into the knee of the plunging ball-carrier. The momentum of the instrumented player increased the counterforce exerted by his head, thereby increasing the resistance to the knee blow. This type of situation did not occur in any of the other four impacts.

By placing force transducers next to each accelerator, we were able not only to measure force but also to get some idea of variable mass (Fig. 5-9). The force curve closely coincided with the linear acceleration curves, indicating that the mass actually varied during the course of a single impact (Fig. 5-10). Simultaneous measurements of force and acceleration allowed us to calculate mass (Fig. 5-11). We found that the human head, which weighs approximately 10 pounds, with well-developed neck musculature, was shown to have an effective mass expressed in pounds ranging from 2 pounds to 490 pounds (Table 5-VI). This additional mass means that the exerted force was significantly greater than the acceleration recordings would indicate.

Holbourn,[4] in a study on gelatin-filled cadaveric heads, concluded that rotational acceleration forces were the main cause of serious injury. He was specifically referring to shear-strain injuries, which result when the brain moves over the rough surfaces of the floor of the skull. The temporal lobes, in the deep recesses of the skull, are likely to be injured in such instances, while the vertex of the brain, with its smooth, overlying bone, and the cerebellum are rarely injured. Impacts to the heads of monkeys, cats, and model heads have demonstrated that supporting the head reduces the incidence of head injury by preventing head rotation.[4,5] Ommaya[8] concluded that the rotational acceleration tolerance of the human brain was about 7,500 radians/sec^2. Because rotational acceleration is associated with most linear accelerations, the injury potential of impact is increased. We were unable to measure rotational acceleration in the concussion-producing impact, but the whiplash effect demonstrated on film indicates rotation very likely did occur.

Linear accelerometers, placed in tangential positions at the periphery of the head, were used to measure tangential accelerations. When this data was combined with a measurement (in inches) of the radius of the player's head, rotational acceleration could then be calculated using the formula $\alpha = \alpha t/r$. It was interesting to note that the tangential accelerations appeared shortly after the linear accelerations, indicating that the first response to a blow is along the line of the blow, with head rotation following thereafter (Fig. 5-12). Results of this investigation are found in Table 5-VII.

The cumulative effect on the brain of repeated blows has been referred to in the literature.[10] During a series of impacts prior to those leading to the concussion-producing play, our instrumented player experienced three high-

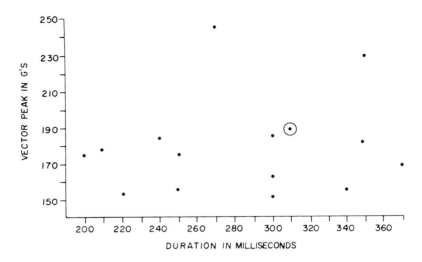

RANGE OF HIGH INTENSITY IMPACTS
NU FOOTBALL SEASON 1970

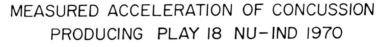

Figure 5-4. A scattergram showing the locations of 15 impacts. The encircled point represents the intensity of the concussion-producing play.

MEASURED ACCELERATION OF CONCUSSION
PRODUCING PLAY 18 NU−IND 1970

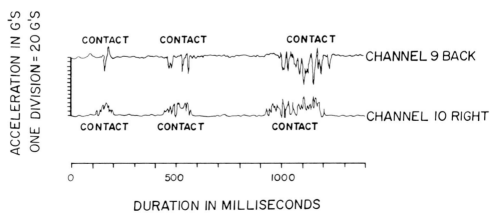

Figure 5-5. Data of concussion-producing play shows two minor impacts and a third high-intensity impact to the left frontal area of the head.

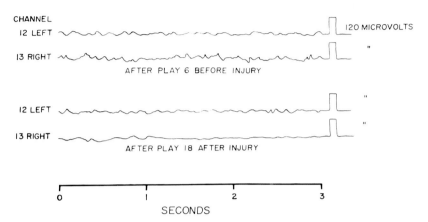

Figure 5-6. Shown above is a telemetered 15 cycle filtered electroencephalogram from each side of the head comparing tracings before and after injury. There is a unilateral decrease in amplitude on the right side of the brain, which persisted.

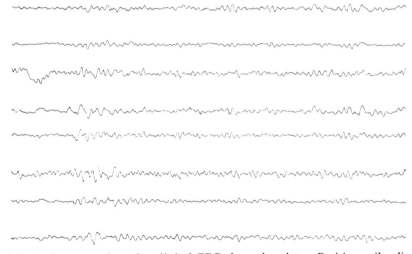

Figure 5-7. An interpretation of a clinical EEG three days later. Positive spike discharges indicate an abnormality with probable locus within the thalamic-hypothalamic region. This type of abnormality is usually seen in adolescence, at times with neurovegetative types of symptoms like headaches and dizzy spells and also at times in patients with behavior disorders. In addition, a very mild slow wave disorder was seen on the frontal occipital and left temporal areas.

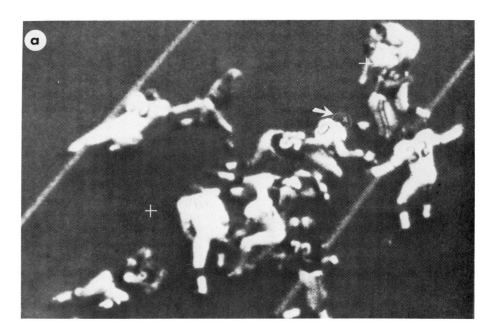

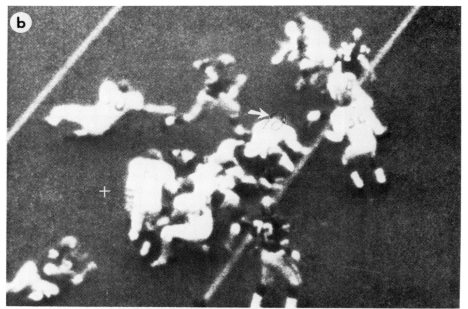

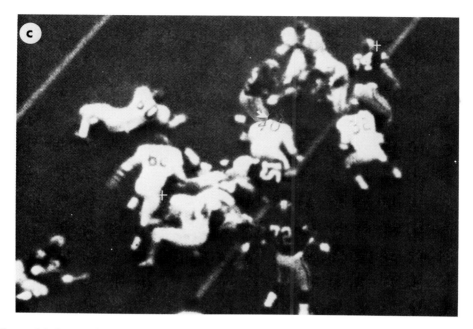

Figure 5-8. Stop action of videotape of concussion-producing play. (a) Player 40 is seen rolling out of block of two opponents, numbers 15 and 44. (b) Shows player further pivoted into approaching ball carrier. (c) The concussion-producing blow may be seen as number 12 strikes the left side of player's head.

intensity impacts in succession. Following these, and despite the fact that there was little evidence of change in the background rhythm of the EEG, the player noted that he felt very fuzzy mentally (Fig. 5-13). Without doubt, the cumulative effect of these earlier three high-intensity impacts, when combined with the four high-intensity impacts immediately preceding the concussion-producing play, could have contributed to the injury that resulted on the fifth impact.

Hollister[5] was the first to report that concussion could be caused in animals by stretching their necks. Conversely, concussion could be prevented when the neck was made rigid through electrical stimulation. Ommaya[8] demonstrated that whiplash without direct head impact produced brain injury in monkeys and that supporting collars could prevent concussion by restraining neck movements. With respect to our injured athlete, cervical cord stretching caused by whiplash during the fifth impact could have contributed to the subsequent concussion by affecting the activity of the reticular core of the brain stem.

Clearly, our telemetry data varied considerably from data obtained in the laboratory under static conditions, leading some investigators to conclude

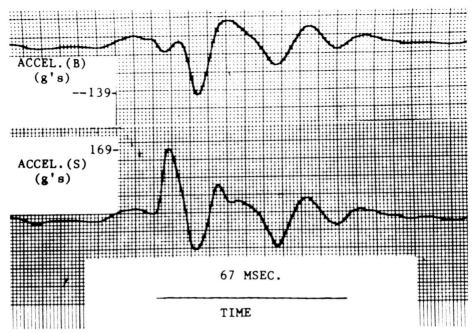

Figure 5-9. Force-time curve showing pounds of force registered on the orthogonally placed linear strain gauges. Courtesy of Appleton-Century-Crofts.

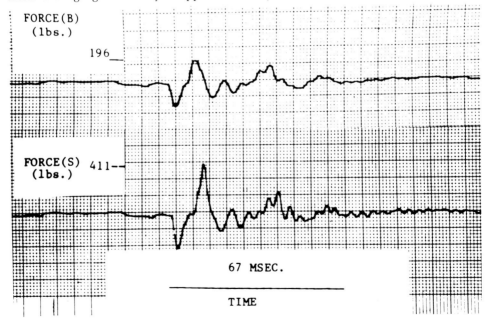

Figure 5-10. Acceleration-time curve resulting from the same impact showing that the accelerations follow the force tracing quite closely. Courtesy of Appleton-Century-Crofts.

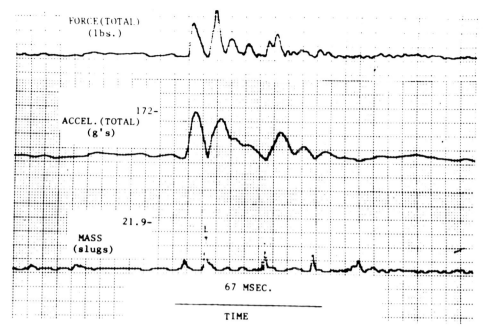

Figure 5-11. Combined curve of force, acceleration, and mass demonstrating that mass varies greatly even during an impact.

Table 5-VI
MEASURED MASSES IN 724 IMPACTS

# On Front of Helmet	Size in Pounds	# On Side of Helmet
48	0– 10	81
94	11– 20	142
110	21– 30	92
80	31– 40	84
44	41– 50	43
38	51– 60	34
30	61– 70	39
36	71– 90	36
31	91–160	35
34	161–260	6
10	261–490	6

that the highest acceleration peak was equal to the effective acceleration and that, in actuality, the human brain could not tolerate this level of effective acceleration for a prolonged period. While the laboratory data consisted of single acceleration peaks with durations of less than ten milliseconds (Fig. 5-14), our data recorded the highest peak of acceleration occurring during

Head and Neck Injuries in Sports

Table 5-VII
PURDUE vs NORTHWESTERN (9-11-76)

Play		Time	Force Vector	Acceleration Vector	Mass in Pounds	Angular Accelerations in Radians/Sec^2
2		60	144.46	124.65	1.15	72
16		160	96.52	50.8	60.8	80
30	(2)	100	73.75	184.66	12.48	65
31	(1)	140	147.51	146.63	32.0	65
31	(3)	5	39.39	41.03	30.72	36
32	(3)	100	125.23	73.23	54.72	21
33	(4)	5	60	14.52	132.16	14
34	(3)	60	216.74	184.66	37.44	65
35	(1)	100	169.81	53.00	102.4	29
35	(2)	60	153.79	41.03	119.68	21
35	(3)	40	216.74	102.59	67.2	36
36	(1)	10	139.94	102.59	43.52	36
36	(2)	40	139.94	102.59	43.52	36
36	(3)	20	139.94	102.59	43.52	36
36	(4)	40	139.94	102.59	43.52	36
37	(2)	40	87.72	41.03	68.16	29
37	(3)	50	149.25	102.59	46.40	36
41		40	96.51	41.03	75.2	21
43	(2)	5	97.67	14.52	215.04	21
44	(3)	60	180.00	66.21	86.72	50
45	(1)	30	102	61.55	52.8	50
45	(2)	60	180	102.59	56.0	65
45	(3)	16	216.74	184.66	37.44	65
46	(1)	5	96.51	33.10	93.12	21
46	(2)	10	165.13	184.66	28.48	65

the entire impact, with duration measured from the onset of acceleration, where the curve left the baseline, and continuing until it finally returned to the baseline and leveled off (Fig. 5-15).

ORIGIN OF ACCELERATION PEAKS

The presence of multiple acceleration peaks in telemetry data indicates that a sudden, sharp resistance occurred serially during the course of an impact. This resistance emanates from the intervertebral joints and spanning ligaments during the stress range of neck motion. It has been shown that seventy-five times more resistance is offered in the stress range than in a normal range of neck motion.[16] Muscles also offer significant resistance during impact, with each muscle acting as a brake for its antagonist, to bring rapid movement to a quick, smooth stop. When tangential acceleration from the quick stretch of neck muscles was recorded, similar acceleration peaks were noted, peaks that were not seen in tracings of linear acceleration.

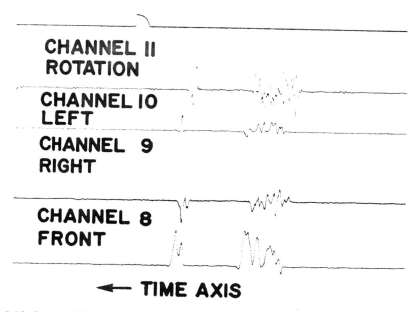

CHANNEL II
ROTATION

CHANNEL 10
LEFT

CHANNEL 9
RIGHT

CHANNEL 8
FRONT

← TIME AXIS

Figure 5-12. Graph of linear and tangential accelerations showing that tangential accelerations occur later than linear accelerations.

Because the electromyographic tracing recorded simultaneously was flat, muscle action could not have been responsible for those multiple peaks (Fig. 5-16). Most likely, then, these peaks in the telemetry recordings resulted from tangential acceleration.

INTERPRETATION OF DATA

Nature of Force

Action on the football field is best described as sustained force. The offensive player sustains his blocks, the defensive player sustains his charge, and the ball carrier sustains a drive to overcome a potential tackler. As a blocker forcefully springs out of his stance, stunning his opponent, his legs immediately coil for further thrusts. Often a charging ball carrier is seemingly stopped at the line until he adds a burst of speed in a second effort, overcoming the resistance and gaining yardage. In such instances, force is added to the initial thrust as resistance is met and overcome. Collisions between football players frequently consist of multiple mini-impacts occurring during a single impact, which explains the prolonged impact periods found in our telemetry data (Figs. 5-19 & 5-20). Figure 5-17 shows four

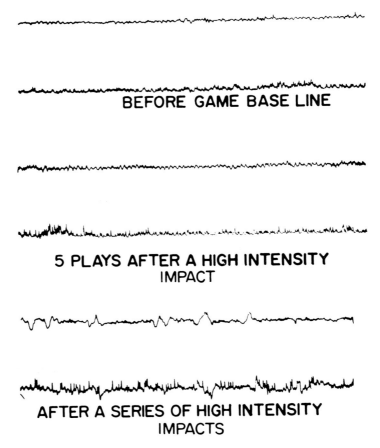

Figure 5-13. Telemetered EEG from the football field showing changes in background rhythm after three successive high-intensity impacts.

individual impacts of a relatively short duration occurring during a single play, while Figure 5-18 shows two impacts of longer duration that occurred in another single play.

Effective Acceleration

The measurement of effective acceleration is difficult when the acceleration-time curve is very irregular (Fig. 5-21). Snyder[13] showed that any peak of acceleration less than four to five milliseconds in duration does not cause injury. Gurdjian[2] increased this time to include impacts of less than ten milliseconds, demonstrating that such impacts have a negligible effect on velocity changes. Vigness[15] also maintained that maximum values of acceleration are significant only when they are of long duration. Versace[14] stated

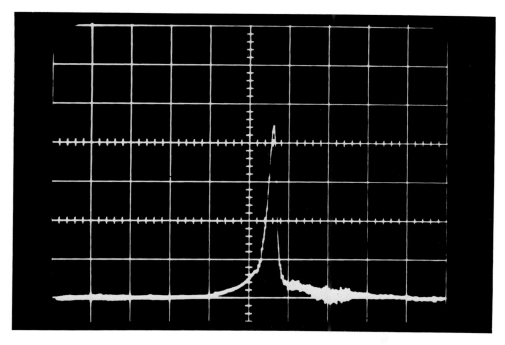

Figure 5-14. Acceleration-time curve of impact to rigid bodies.

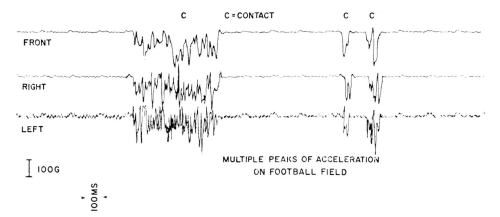

Figure 5-15. Telemetered graph of impact on the football field.

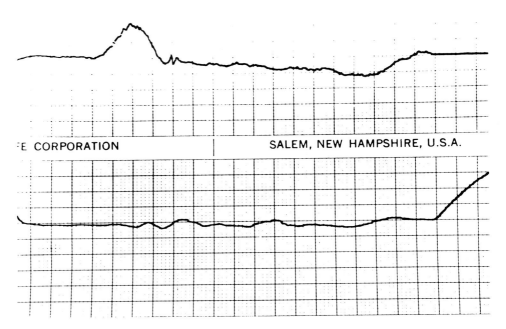

Figure 5-16. Graph of quick stretch of neck muscles of an athlete showing resultant accelerations in the upper graph and a flat EMG in the lower graph resulting from a surprise drop of a weight in the laboratory. Courtesy of Appleton-Century-Crofts.

that the effective acceleration in a grossly irregular tracing is somewhat greater than one-half of the peak values. Regardless of the source of these multiple peaks, however, and even if they prove to be artifactual as some investigators maintain, these peaks play a minor role in causing injury on the football field and thus can be ignored.

Versace devised a method of measuring the effective acceleration from a graph of a grossly irregular response.[14] Using this method to measure the effective acceleration of the concussion-producing play, the effective acceleration worked out to be 80 G's despite a single peak of 188 G's measured during the play. The figure of 80 G's was arrived at by ignoring that part of the peak that had a duration of less than 5 milliseconds. The effective acceleration for the entire response was one-half the amplitude of the remaining parts of the peaks.

Although we encountered no further injuries to the instrumented player for the remainder of our study, we continued to obtain telemetry data, which is presented in Tables 5-VIII, 5-IX, and 5-X.

Duration of Telemetered Impacts

Our telemetry studies have demonstrated that the duration of impacts on the football field lasts nearly 40 times longer than that of simulated impacts conducted under laboratory conditions. Initially, this statement appears highly questionable, since the force involved in, for example, a flying tackle, where a player propels himself off his feet and into his opponent, would probably not last 40 milliseconds, even with the opponent resisting to his maximum (Fig. 5-22). The concept of sustained force explains this seeming contradiction.

In impacts on the football field, the force involved does not occur in one short, powerful burst. Rather, the initial force is sustained, with more effort being continually added to sustain the initial force. During the total impact time as energy is being absorbed, additional energy is being expended. We have provided a formula for converting energy to force in the Appendix so that this concept can be more easily understood. Essentially, during a prolonged response, several successive and overlapping mini-impacts of varying levels of acceleration occur.

SUMMARY

The multiple variables involved in a single impact on the football field make it impossible to calculate the exact maximums for brain tolerance before injury will result. Our telemetry studies did prove conclusively, however, that the range of values for maximum brain tolerance obtained by other investigators under laboratory conditions cannot be compared to the values measured on the football field. The reason for the difference between the laboratory data and our telemetry data is that the static conditions of the laboratory cannot reproduce the variables found on the field. Specifically, there is no way to duplicate in the laboratory the phenomenon of energy absorption that occurs during the collision of two players as a result of a *sustained type* of force. Truly, therefore, any reliable range of values for the tolerance of the brain to impact will not come from laboratory experiments but, rather, from data collected from actual impacts, such as those occurring on the football field between human beings.

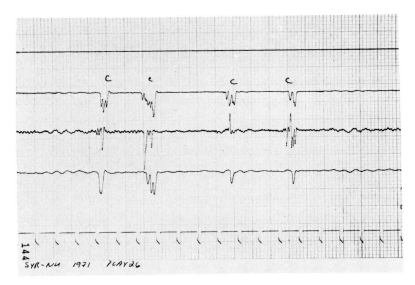

Figure 5-17. Four individual impacts occurring during a single play.

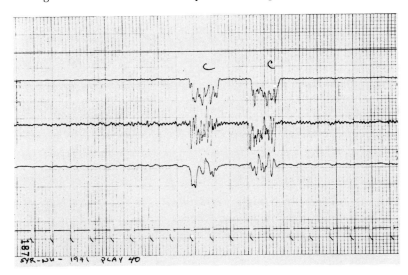

Figure 5-18. Two individual impacts of longer duration that occur during a single play.

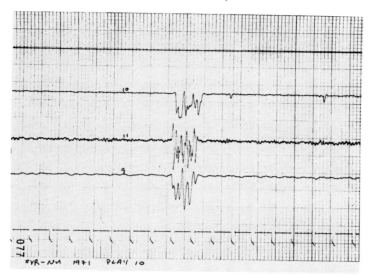

Figure 5-19. A single impact occurring during a single play.

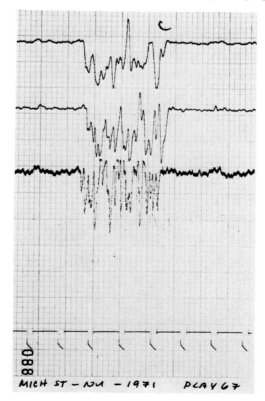

Figure 5-20. A large single impact, probably a combination of several impacts of short duration.

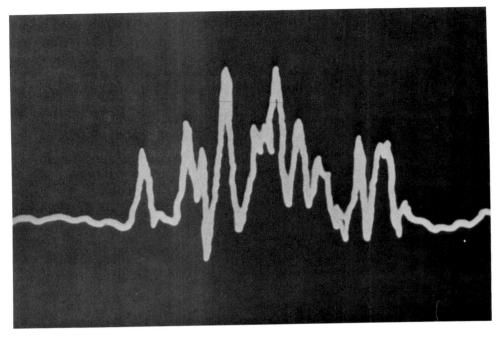

Figure 5-21. Very irregular acceleration-time curve.

Table 5-VIII
NORTH CAROLINA vs NORTHWESTERN (9-18-76)

Play		Time	Average Force in Pounds		Vector	Average Accel. in G's		Vector	Mass in G's		Mass in Pounds
			Front	Side		Front	Side		Front	Side	
2		40	86	91	125.2	123	72	142.52	.69	1.26	40.32
4	(1)	10	69	55	88.23	13	29	31.78	2.37	1.89	75.84
4	(2)	40	155	164	225.65	123	72	142.52	1.26	2.27	72.64
5		80	172	146	225.61	55	96	110.63	3.12	1.52	99.84
6		60	69	91	114.2	55	43	69.81	1.25	2.11	67.52
7		100	86	73	112.8	27	57	63.07	3.18	1.28	101.76
10		80	103	73	126.24	27	42	49.92	3.81	1.73	121.92
11	(1)	20	69	110	129.84	41	14	43.32	1.68	7.85	251.20
11	(2)	40	86	146	169.44	68	72	99.03	1.26	2.02	64.64
12		40	86	55	102.08	55	57	79.2	1.56	.96	49.92
14	(1)	80	69	36	77.82	13	14	43.32	5.3	2.57	169.60
14	(2)	40	103	55	116.76	68	42	79.92	1.51	1.3	48.32
15	(1)	40	103	73	126.24	96	57	111.64	1.07	1.28	40.96
15	(2)	80	87	128	154.76	109	129	168.88	.79	.99	31.68
16	(1)	60	69	55	88.23	13	14	43.32	5.3	3.92	169.60
16	(2)	100	137	91	164.46	27	57	63.07	5.07	1.59	162.24
17	(1)	20	69	36	77.82	13	14	43.32	5.3	2.57	169.60
17	(2)	80	86	55	102.08	27	28	38.89	3.18	1.96	101.76
18	(1)	40	69	55	88.23	13	28	30.87	5.3	1.96	169.60
18	(2)	120	206	164	263.3	41	86	95.27	5.02	1.9	160.64
18	(3)	100	86	73	112.8	27	42	49.92	3.18	1.73	101.76
19		80	86	55	102.08	27	42	49.92	3.18	1.3	101.76
20		40	69	58	90.13	13	14	43.32	5.3	4.14	196.60

Table 5-IX
NORTH CAROLINA vs NORTHWESTERN (9-18-76)

Play		Time	Average Force in Pounds		Vector	Average Accel. in G's		Vector	Mass in G's		Mass in Pounds
			Front	Side		Front	Side		Front	Side	
21		20	34	18	38.47	13	14	43.32	2.61	1.28	83.52
22		60	120	18	121.34	13	28	30.87	9.23	.64	295.36
23	(1)	40	86	73	112.8	55	42	69.2	1.56	1.73	55.36
23	(2)	80	172	146	225.61	109	101	148.6	1.57	1.44	50.24
23	(3)	40	86	91	125.2	40	86	94.84	.94	1.05	33.60
26		80	103	73	126.24	27	42	49.92	3.81	1.73	121.92
30	(1)	20	69	91	114.2	27	42	49.92	2.55	2.16	81.60
30	(2)	20	87	55	102.92	13	14	19.10	6.69	3.92	214.08
30	(3)	60	103	55	116.76	13	28	30.87	7.92	1.96	253.44
31	(1)	120	51	36	62.42	13	14	19.10	3.92	2.57	125.44
31	(2)	40	51	36	62.42	13	14	19.10	3.92	2.57	125.44
31	(4)	60	103	73	126.24	13	28	30.87	7.92	2.6	253.44
32	(1)	80	17	18	24.75	13	14	19.10	1.3	1.28	41.60
32	(2)	40	17	37	24.75	13	14	19.10	1.3	2.64	84.48
33	(2)	60	120	91	150.6	27	42	49.92	4.44	2.16	142.08
34	(1)	40	154	73	170.42	82	42	92.13	1.87	1.73	59.84
34	(2)	60	86	73	112.8	13	28	30.87	6.61	2.6	211.52
34	(3)	40	172	73	186.85	123	72	142.52	1.39	1.01	44.48
35		60	87	55	102.92	13	29	31.78	6.69	1.89	214.08
36		40	69	128	145.41	96	115	149.8	.71	1.11	35.52
37		60	103	55	116.76	13	29	31.78	7.92	1.89	253.44
38	(1)	60	69	36	77.82	13	14	19.10	5.3	2.57	169.60
39	(4)	20	34	18	38.47	13	14	19.10	2.61	1.28	29.39

Table 5-X
NORTH CAROLINA vs NORTHWESTERN (9-18-76)

Play		Time	Average Force in Pounds		Vector	Average Accel. in G's		Vector	Mass in G's		Mass in Pounds
			Front	Side		Front	Side		Front	Side	
40		60	69	55	88.23	13	29	31.78	5.3	1.89	169.60
41	(1)	60	69	110	129.84	55	129	140.23	1.25	.85	40
41	(2)	40	87	55	102.92	13	29	31.78	6.69	1.89	214.08
41	(3)	40	51	91	104.31	82	158	178.01	.62	.57	19.84
41	(5)	60	103	55	116.76	13	29	31.78	7.92	1.89	253.44
42	(1)	40	87	55	102.92	13	14	19.10	6.69	3.92	214.08
42	(2)	80	172	91	194.58	96	115	149.8	1.79	.79	57.28
42	(3)	60	103	73	126.24	13	29	31.78	7.92	2.51	253.44
42	(4)	40	34	91	97.14	13	14	19.10	2.61	6.5	208
42	(5)	40	120	18	121.34	109	14	109.89	1.1	1.28	40.96
42	(9)	66	51	55	75.0	13	14	19.1	3.92	3.92	125.44
42	(10)	60	137	113	177.58	41	43	59.41	3.34	2.62	106.88
42	(11)	60	120	73	140.45	13	29	31.78	9.23	2.51	295.36
43	(1)	60	51	164	171.74	82	86	118.82	.62	1.90	60.80
43	(2)	140	103	110	150.69	96	43	105.19	1.07	2.55	81.60
43	(3)	80	86	73	112.8	82	72	109.12	1.04	1.01	33.28
44	(1)	60	69	55	88.23	13	29	31.78	5.3	1.89	169.60
44	(2)	40	172	91	194.58	41	129	135.35	4.19	.70	134.08
45	(1)	40	103	91	137.44	41	58	71.02	2.51	1.56	80.32
45	(2)	40	86	146	169.44	68	101	121.75	1.26	1.44	46.08
45	(3)	60	137	146	200.21	68	72	99.03	2.01	2.02	64.64
46	(1)	100	137	110	175.69	150	129	197.84	.91	.85	29.12
46	(4)	80	154	110	189.25	96	144	173.06	1.6	.76	51.20
47		40	137	110	175.69	115	115	162.63	1.19	.95	38.08

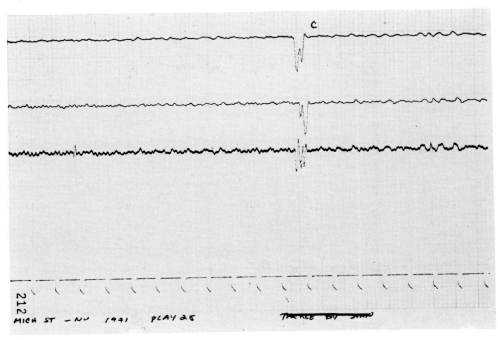

Figure 5-22. This type of acceleration graph was produced if the player left his feet in a flying tackle.

REFERENCES

1. Gold, A. J., Hance, H. E., Kornhauser, M., and Lawton, R. W.: Impact tolerance of restrained mice as a function of velocity change and average deceleration. *Aerospace Med, 33*:204, 1962.

2. Gurdjian, E. S., Roberts, V. L., and Thomas, L. M.: Tolerance curves of acceleration and intracranial pressure and protective index in experimental head injury. *J Trauma, 6*:600, 1966.

3. Henneman, E.: Organization of the motor system—a preview. In Mountcastle, V. B.: *Medical Physiology,* 13th ed. St. Louis, Mosby, 1974, p. 603.

4. Holbourn, A. H.: Mechanics of head injuries. *Lancet, 2*:438, 1943.

5. Hollister, N. R., Jolley, W. P., and Horne, P. G.: Biophysics of concussion. Part I, WADC Technical Report 58-193, *ASTIA Document* #AD203385, Sept., 1958.

6. Hughes, J. R., Wilms, J. H., Adams, C. L., and Combs, L. W.: Football helmet evaluation based on players' EEG's. *The Physician & Sports Medicine,* May, 1977, p 73.

7. Lissner, H. R., Lebow, M., and Evans, F. G.: Experimental studies on relation between acceleration and intracranial pressure changes in man. *Surg Gynecol & Obstet, 111*:329, 1960.

8. Ommaya, A. K., Faas, F., and Yarnell, P.: Whiplash injury and brain damage: an experimental study. *JAMA, 204*:285, 1968.

9. Reid, S. E., Tarkington, J. A., Epstein, H. E., and O'Dea, T. J.: Brain tolerance to impact in football. *Surg Gynecol & Obstet, 133*:929, 1971.

10. Roberts, A. H.: Brain damage in boxing. In *Brain Damage in Sport* London, 1969. (Quoted in *Lancet,* Feb. 21, 1976, p. 400.)

11. Rushmer, R. F., Green, E. L., and Kingsley, H. D.: Internal injuries produced by abrupt deceleration of experimental animals. *J Aviat Med, 17*:511, 1946.

12. Shaw, J. C.: A method for continuously recording characteristics of EEG topography. *Electroencephalogr Clin Neurophysiol, 29*:592, 1970.

13. Snyder, R. G.: Human impact tolerance. *International Automobile Conference Compendium* #700398, Society of Automotive Engineers, 1970, p. 728.

14. Versace, J.: Review of severity index. *Proceedings of the 15th Stapp Car Crash Conference.* Warrendale, PA: Society of Automotive Engineers, 1971, p. 771.

15. Vigness, I.: Shock motions and their management. *Exp Mech, 1*:1319, 1961.

16. White, A. A., III, and Panjabi, M. M.: *Clinical Biomechanics of the Spine.* Philadelphia, Lippincott, 1978, p. 23.

Chapter 6

MECHANISMS OF INJURY

The head and neck of an athlete who participates in contact sports must be able to absorb impacts of high intensity. Consider this: a helmet that can tolerate no more than 80 foot-pounds of energy in the laboratory can be subjected to over 37 times as much energy on the football field! It has been demonstrated that a 224-pound player, running at full speed, can deliver over 3,000 foot-pounds of energy at the moment of collision with another player. It becomes evident, therefore, that the helmet can provide only partial protection from head and neck injuries; the remainder of this protection must be supplied by the defensive responses of the player. Before we discuss the mechanisms of injury and how such injuries may be prevented, a brief review of the anatomy and physiology of the head and neck is necessary.

ANATOMY AND PHYSIOLOGY

Skull

The human skull, or cranium, is an irregularly shaped, heterogeneous bony shell. The floor is rough due to the bony ridges dividing the surface into the anterior, medial, and posterior recesses (Fig. 6-1), while the ceiling of the cranium is perfectly smooth. The foramen magnum is the large opening in the base of the skull through which the spinal cord passes.

Bony Spine

A typical cervical vertebra is composed of the following parts: (1) the body, the weight-bearing block of bone in front of the cord; (2) the bony arch, which projects posteriorly, encircling and protecting the cord; and (3) three projections extending from the arch on which the muscles pull (i.e. the spinous process, projecting posteriorly, and two transverse processes, which project laterally on the right and left) (Fig. 6-2). That part of the bony arch extending from the body to the transverse process is referred to as the pedicle, while the remainder of the arch, which extends from each transverse process to the spinous process, is the lamina. A notch on the superior and inferior surface of each pedicle forms an exit between adjacent vertebrae for the peripheral nerve roots. This exit is called the intervertebral foramen.

ANTERIOR

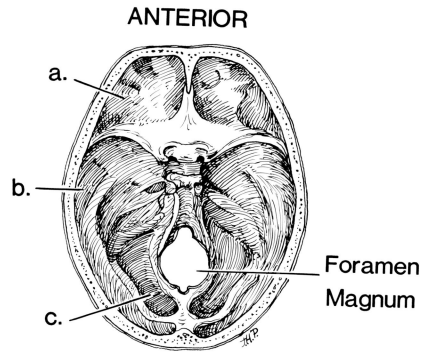

Figure 6-1. An illustration of the skull floor showing the uneven surface due to the anterior, middle, and posterior fossae.

Each vertebra is joined to its neighbor by a right and left articular process extending above and below to similar processes on adjacent vertebrae. These four-faceted projections form faceted joints, which are secured by capsules and ligaments that function to prevent forward displacement of an upper vertebra on a lower one. These joints are not normally weight bearing, but they do limit movement between two adjacent vertebrae and, as such, act as bony stops and ligaments. It is important to note that the first and second cervical vertebrae are highly specialized and differ from the five remaining cervical vertebrae in that they have neither definite bodies nor intervertebral discs between them.

The adult vertebral column viewed laterally reveals four normal curves: convex anteriorly in the cervical and lumbar regions and convex posteriorly in the thoracic and sacral regions. The curvature of the spine gives the spinal column increased flexibility and shock-absorbing capacity (Fig. 6-3).

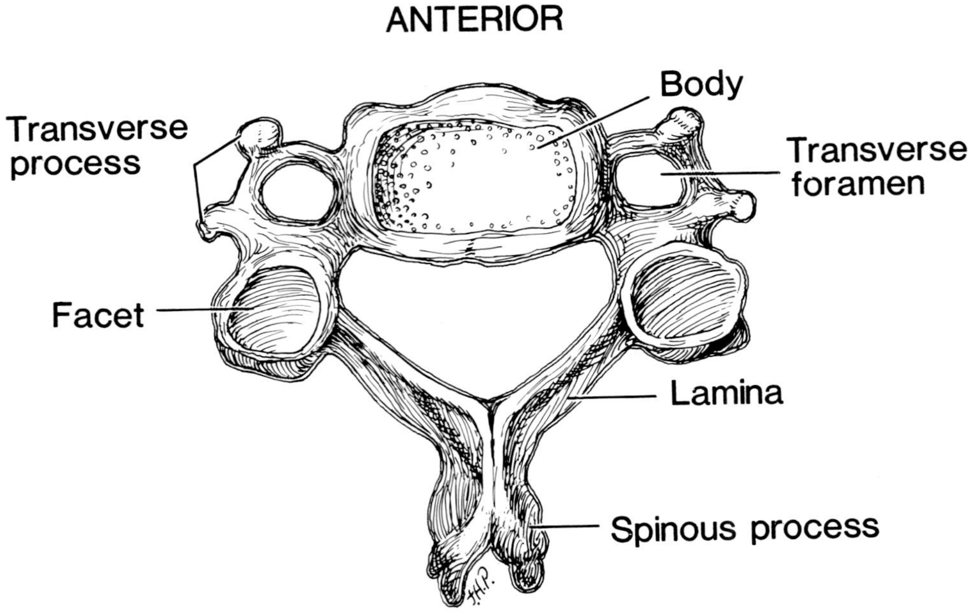

Head and Neck Injuries in Sports

ANTERIOR

Body

Transverse process

Transverse foramen

Facet

Lamina

Spinous process

Figure 6-2. Shown is typical cervical vertebra as seen from above. The bifid spinous process and the foramen in the transverse process for passage of the vertebral artery are identifying features of the cervical vertebrae.

Intervertebral Discs

The intervertebral discs are fibrocartilaginous structures that completely fill the spaces between the bodies of the vertebrae. The disc consists of an outer annulus fibrosus that is composed of concentric, laminated bands with crisscrossing fibers. The arrangement of diagonal fibers in the annulus fibrosus provides little resistance to the distortion of its shape as a result of the varied stresses within the normal range of motion, but it does exert great resistance beyond this range. The center of the disc is the nucleus pulposus, which is composed of a loose network of fine fibrous bands surrounded by a gel having a water content of 70 percent to 90 percent. The nucleus is the pivotal point of all spine motion, enduring much of the stress applied to the spine. The discs blend into the bodies of the vertebrae and into the anterior and posterior longitudinal ligaments. They bulge anteriorly in flexion, posteriorly in extension, and toward the concavity of the spinal curve in lateral bending. Normal discs tolerate more of the stress of crushing loads than do the bodies of the vertebrae.

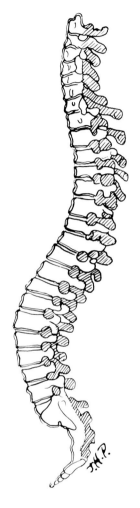

Figure 6-3. The normal curvatures of the entire human spine absorb some of the shock of compression blows.

Ligaments

Ligaments are thin, tough, fibrous bands of varying widths that span the bony joints and restrict motion by their firm attachment to the bone on either side of a joint. The large amounts of energy that are exerted during traumatic situations are absorbed by a counterforce exerted by the ligaments protecting a particular joint. Ligaments, unlike muscle, are relatively inactive; they stretch and contract very little.

Great ranges of neck motion involve many individual joints; therefore, several ligaments are required to restrict this motion. Three primary ligaments perform this function in combination with several specialized short ligaments that unite the skull and the first two cervical vertebrae, and with individual ligaments connecting each of the three bony projections on a vertebra with their counterparts on adjacent vertebrae. The anterior longitudinal ligament is an important ligament in limiting neck motion (Fig. 6-4). It extends from the skull and attaches to all vertebral bodies and intervertebral discs, thereby covering the entire anterior aspect of the bodies of the vertebrae. Another main ligament is the posterior longitudinal ligament, which connects the posterior surface of the bodies of the vertebrae. This ligament is narrower and weaker than its counterpart, which runs in front of the vertebral bodies, but it is nonetheless firmly attached to the discs and protects the anterior aspect of the spinal cord. Probably the most important of the three major ligaments is the *ligamentum flavum*. This ligament is unique in that it contains a large amount of elastic tissue that permits it to stretch to 15 percent of its length and thereby preventing buckling when the neck is extended.[20] Fibers of this ligament extend from the anterior-inferior border of the lamina above to the posterior-superior border of the lamina below, allowing some tilting of the posterior bony arch and steadying each lamina. The fibers in the ligaments extending from the bony projections of the vertebrae are arranged in a diagonal manner to permit some give, but they are basically inactive structures. The faceted joints of the cervical spine have loose capsules to permit normal range of motion (Fig. 6-5). Movement at these joints below C_2 is that of a gliding motion on the vertebra below.

Muscles

Seven deep muscles located along the anterior aspect of the neck have segmental attachments to the cervical vertebrae and support the function of the spanning sternocleidomastoid muscle in resisting forced extension of the neck.[2,12] Four of these muscles lie medial to all the branches of the brachial plexus; the remaining three muscles are located laterally to these peripheral nerves. The powerful paravertebral muscles and the trapezius muscle at the back of the neck resist forced flexion of the neck.

Muscle response can be understood by examining the reaction of paired muscles. A particular muscle is most closely related to its direct antagonist, such as the biceps and triceps. When either of the pair shortens, the opposing muscle lengthens. Direct antagonists are of great importance because precise control of movements frequently involves application of a braking action, and each muscle in a pair acts as a brake for its antagonist, serving to bring rapid movement to a quick, smooth stop.[4,1] Recordings of electrical activity of a muscle and its antagonist reveal that during a contraction of a muscle, there is usually some activity in its antagonist. Toward the end of a rapid contraction, this activity increases sharply.

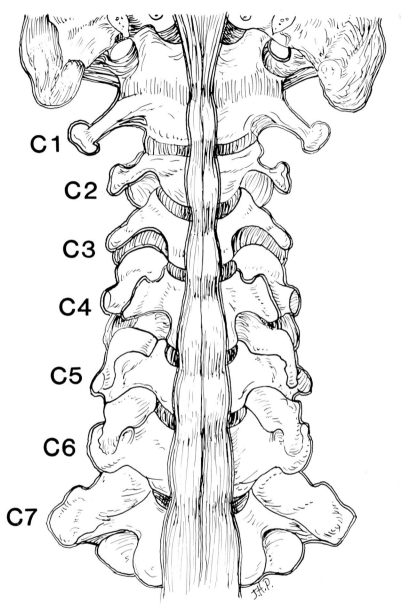

C1

C2

C3

C4

C5

C6

C7

Figure 6-4. Anterior longitudinal ligament firmly adherent to the anterior surfaces of the bodies of vertebrae aligns the spine when taut in slight extension of the neck.

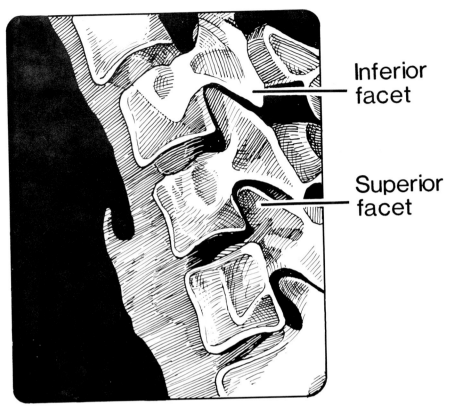

Figure 6-5. Faceted joints of cervical spine showing what is seen on lateral x-ray view of the neck.

Central Nervous System

The central nervous system, which includes the brain and spinal cord, floats in cerebrospinal fluid. A closed hydraulic system is thereby formed, which is contained by an envelope of three membranes, called meninges, enclosing the brain and spinal cord. The dura mater is a tough, fibrous membrane attached directly to the skull, forming a covering for the delicate second membrane, the arachnoid mater. The inner pia mater completely covers the brain and cord like skin. The cerebrospinal fluid circulates nutrients to the entire nervous system and provides a cushion for the brain and spinal cord. This fluid completely fills the subarachnoid space between the arachnoid and pia mater, pressing the arachnoid against the dura mater so that only a potential subdural space is left. The inner layer of the dura mater partially subdivides the cranial cavity into compartments. This prevents shifting of the brain and forms venous sinuses from folds in the membrane for the drainage of blood from the meningeal veins.

The Brain

The human brain, having about the same consistency of gelatin, readily conforms to changes in the configuration of the skull caused by impact. The brain is divided anatomically into the forebrain, midbrain, and hindbrain. The forebrain is the largest section and is principally composed of the two large cerebral hemispheres. The midbrain, a short, cylindrical structure, connects the forebrain with the spinal cord. The hindbrain includes the cerebellum, the pons, and the medulla oblongata. The cerebellum controls and regulates muscular movement, the pons connects the two lobes of the cerebellum, and the medulla—the center for reflex activity and respiration—is the upward continuation of the spinal cord. The brain stem includes the midbrain and hindbrain, excluding the cerebellum and pons.

Spinal Cord

The spinal cord begins where the brain stem ends and is housed in the spinal canal. Its thickness varies, being the greatest in the cervical spine, which has a thickness of about the tip of the little finger. The cord is protected by the bony canal, which has a diameter about twice that of the cord.

Peripheral Nerves

The anterior, or motor, and posterior, or sensory, nerve roots leave the cervical spine together through the intervertebral foramina and immediately separate. The anterior roots unite to form peripheral nerve plexuses.

The cervical plexus, formed by the upper four cervical roots, supplies sensation to the head and face. The greater occipital nerve formed from the C_2 segment emerges through muscles at the base of the skull and supplies sensation to the back and top of the head.

The brachial plexus, formed from the lower four cervical roots and first thoracic segment, provides innervation to the muscles of the entire upper extremity (Fig. 6-6).

C_5 plus C_6—shoulder girdle and upper arm
C_5—deltoid muscle (axillary nerve)
C_5—biceps muscle, etc. (musculocutaneous nerve)
C_6—triceps muscle (radial nerve)
C_7 plus C_8—controls movements of wrist and fingers
C_7—extension (radial nerve)

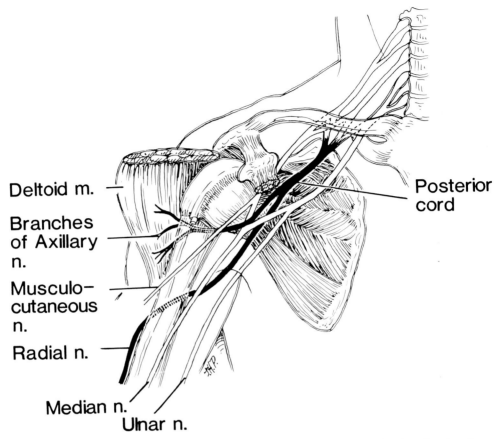

Deltoid m.

Branches
of Axillary
n.

Musculo-
cutaneous
n.

Radial n.

Median n.

Ulnar n.

Posterior
cord

Figure 6-6. Brachial plexus with emphasis of the posterior cord and showing the circuitous route of the axillary nerve wrapped around the posterior surface of the neck of the humerus to supply the deltoid muscle.

C_8—flexion (median nerve)
T_1—intrinsic muscles of the hand (median and ulnar nerves)

The spinal cord is more firmly fixed to the bony cervical spine than to the thoracic or lumbar spine. The nerves of the brachial plexus follow a relatively straight course through the neck, emerging with the subclavian artery between the clavicle and the first rib in a cleft formed by the anterior and middle scalene muscles. The posterior cord of the brachial plexus sends a branch, the axillary nerve, to the deltoid and teres minor muscles. This nerve, after leaving the posterior cord, winds posteriorly around the neck of the humerus to supply the deltoid muscle and the overlying skin.

RANGE OF MOTION

Due to the smaller-sized vertebrae in the neck, the cervical spine has the greatest range of motion of the entire human spine. This range of motion includes flexion, extension, lateral flexion, and rotation in all directions. Most movements of the cervical spine, however, combine rotation with flexion or extension.

Range of motion is divided into three categories: normal range, stress range, and trauma range (Fig. 6-7). Within the normal range there is smooth movement at each of the eight cervical joints, movement that is limited by the ligaments guarding the joint. During normal movement only natural resistance resulting from inertia and the compressive action of the intervertebral discs restrict motion. It should be noted here that there is significantly less resistance in flexion of the cervical spine than there is in extension.

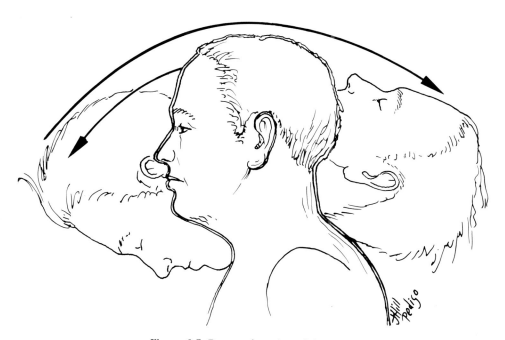

Figure 6-7. Range of motion of the neck.

The normal position of the cervical spine is that of slight extension. Flexion at the junction between the occiput and the first cervical vertebra, extending from full extension to full flexion, spans an angle of about 45 degrees. Most of the flexion and extension in the cervical spine below this level occurs between C_3 to C_7, with a maximum at C_5 to C_6 of 17 degrees.

Lateral flexion occurs at about the mid-portion of the cervical spine and is restricted to about 11 degrees. The maximum rotation in this area occurs at the joint between C_1 and C_2, encompassing an arc of about 47 degrees. Rotation in the mid-cervical area is only about 12 degrees.[21,12]

PRINCIPLES OF INJURY

In order to change the speed or direction of an object in motion or to move a body at rest, force is required. If there is no resistance to motion, there is no force. When one football player exerts a force on a second player during a collision, the second player simultaneously exerts a counterforce upon the first player. These forces are equal in magnitude but are opposite in direction. Either force may be considered the action and the other the reaction. Even though either or both players may be injured in a given impact (depending upon how the blow is delivered and received), we will assume here that the defensive player is responsible for the resultant injury and will concentrate on how he reacts to the impact. We will also limit the extent of injury to the head and neck, although the same principles apply to injury to any part of the body. Momentum will be used to describe the energy of the offensive player; the term counterforce will refer to the resistance of the defensive player during a collision.

The impulse-momentum theorum ($Ft = \Delta MV$) describes the mechanics involved in any given collision. The mass (M) of the offensive player multiplied by his velocity (V) equals his momentum. Momentum is changed (Δ) (that is, reduced, stopped, or increased) in a collision by a force (F) applied over a certain period of time (t) by the defensive player. The time required to change momentum is inversely proportional to the amount of force used to effect this change: less force is required when resistance is applied over a prolonged period of time; greater force is necessary to produce a momentum change over a brief period of time. Whether or not injury will occur depends on four variables: (1) momentum, (2) the degree of resistance, (3) the direction of the blow and its impact point on the player's body, and (4) the structural strength of the player.

In sports that do not involve vehicles, momentum is limited by the weight of the athlete, which rarely exceeds 300 pounds, and the velocity, which is approximately 30 feet per second.

Resisting the advance of the ball is the goal of the defense in football; the aim of the offense is to overcome this resistance. Injury will occur at either of the two extremes of offered resistance: (1) when unyielding resistance is offered and (2) when no resistance is offered. Unyielding resistance in its truest sense is the resistance of an immobile structure with a hard surface, such as the bottom of a swimming pool, and it is easy to understand why injury would occur upon impact with such a structure. Injury can also occur when there is too little resistance to a blow, causing the head to be driven beyond its normal range of motion.

The direction of the blow and its impact point on the player's body is a significant factor in determining injury potential. If the blow is delivered to the top of the head and directed along the axis of the spine, injury can result from compression of the bodies of the vertebrae upon one another. A blow delivered along the axis of the spine in the opposite direction tends to pull the vertebrae apart, and great tensile strength is required in order to avoid a disruptive type of injury. A blow delivered at right angles to the axis of the spine produces shearing forces that strain ligaments and tend to knock one vertebra out of alignment with an adjoining vertebral body. Very few blows are aligned perfectly with the cervical spine; most blows, in fact, strike off center, introducing an element of rotation to flexion or extension as the body moves in an altered direction.

Finally, the structural strength of the neck is of particular importance in determining injury potential. The vertebral bodies are composed of soft, cancellous bone, with a thin covering of cortical bone. They can absorb some energy as they are compressed by the axial blow, but they are more easily injured by compressive forces than are either the discs or the hard cortical bone that forms the bony arch and articular processes. Actually, it is the ligaments that provide the tensile strength of the neck. Roaf[14] found that the anterior and posterior longitudinal ligaments are rarely injured in pure hyperextension of the cervical spine, however, when the variable of rotation is added, these ligaments can be more easily ruptured. This principle can be demonstrated by tearing a piece of adhesive tape. A straight pull along the axis of its fibers will not tear the tape because all fibers are resisting simultaneously. However, when stress is applied to the edge of the tape, single fibers are torn individually and successively until the entire width of the tape is torn. Normal rotation under these circumstances is restricted by muscle action, demonstrating the dynamic action of muscles that react when needed to prevent injury to ligaments.

MECHANISMS OF INJURY

When an external force is exerted, it can cause structural failure to an immobile head or it can cause movement of the head and neck beyond the normal range and into the stress range of motion, causing stretching of ligaments and compression of discs and bony structures. During the stress range, resistance is seventy-five times greater than it is in the normal range, and nearly seven times more energy is absorbed by these structures.[20] In the trauma range of motion, the external force exceeds the resistance of the head and neck, resulting in structural failure.

It has been demonstrated on the playing field that injury is more likely to occur when a blow is delivered at some unguarded moment, such as after the referee's whistle has signaled the end of the play or when a ball carrier steps out of bounds. During this time muscles are relaxed, and the neck passes through its normal range of motion and into the stress and trauma range with very little offered resistance. Impacts under these conditions occur in such a brief time period that muscle reflexes are incapable of responding. Injury results because no voluntary resistance is offered to reduce the momentum of the blow or to prolong the time the neck travels through its ranges of motion.

Skull Injuries

Structural injury to the skull results from deformation forces that exceed the tensile strength of the structure. The skull is rarely injured in football because of the protection afforded by the modern helmet. Injury can occur, however, when the helmet is lost during a play or where the head is inadequately protected, such as in sandlot games. Sports involving missiles, such as baseball, golf, or track, can cause skull injuries, as in the case of a pitched ball that strikes the head of a batter or a line drive that hits a pitcher who is temporarily off balance after throwing the ball. Injury is likely in such a situation because the baseball delivers a great force to a small area of the skull, as measured in pounds per square inch. It has been determined that 580 inch-pounds of energy generated by a pitched ball can cause a skull fracture.[5] In this instance, the skull would be deformed by the blow, with an indentation in the region of the impact accompanied by an outbending of the skull at the periphery of the indented portion. Fracture occurs when the deformation exceeds the tensile strength of the skull. A linear fracture may occur at the periphery of the indented area, or if sufficient force has been delivered to this area, a depressed skull fracture results. Because the vault of the skull is more elastic and convex, it can withstand sudden distortion; however, the base of the skull is rigid and, therefore, more vulnerable to injury. A basal skull fracture can occur, for example, in a skater who strikes the back of his head in a fall to the ice. This fracture, and those fractures that occur over the frontal sinus in the supraorbital area, involves air sinuses and is considered to be a compound fracture, carrying the added risk of infection. The middle meningeal artery lies in a groove in the inner table of the temporal bone in front of the ear. A linear skull fracture crossing this groove may injure this vessel and result in severe brain hemorrhage.[16]

Cervical Spine Injuries

Injuries of the cervical spine can range from a mild sprain of ligaments surrounding the intervertebral joints to fractures and dislocations of the cervical vertebrae as these components pass through their various ranges of motion. The degree of resistance offered by the intact cervical spine determines the type of injury. The athlete who strikes his opponent with the crown of his helmet has aligned his cervical spine in the direction of the blow. In this position he cannot see the oncoming opponent and is, therefore, unable to make any adjustments to the blow. Should the blow be directed along the axis of his spine, great resistance would be offered by his rigid cervical spine during a very brief period of impact. The result will be a severe compressive blow, with the bony spine subjected to great stress. A fracture of the first cervical vertebra is possible, or in the lower cervical spine, where articular facets and discs are stronger than the vertebral body, varying degrees of compression of vertebral bodies may occur, depending upon the momentum of the blow. Such compression may result in injuries ranging from a chip fracture of the anterior border to an actual wedging of the entire portion of the body, forcing the spine into flexion and producing a jackknife injury as the force continues to hyperflex the cervical spine. Since the entire stress of the blow is taken by the bodies of the vertebra, a serious Type IV teardrop injury[17] results in which the vertebra is crushed and forced posteriorly, injuring the cord as the faceted joints are disrupted, rupturing the disc and fracturing the laminae. The mechanisms involved in this type of injury may be better understood by using the example of a man in an upright position who jumps from a four-foot table. If his knees were extended and locked on landing, serious injury could result, since the full blow would be absorbed by his bony skeleton. By simply bending his knees before landing, which would allow his quadriceps muscles to bring him to a stop over a longer period of time, he would take the pressure off the bony joints and would land safely.

An equally serious injury occurs when a player with his head in a flexed position strikes an opponent so that the blow forces the neck into extreme flexion. This results in a compressive hyperflexion injury as the lower cervical spine is forced into the trauma range of flexion. In this type of injury, the force continues to compress the bodies of the fifth and sixth cervical vertebrae, forcing them posteriorly into the spinal cord. This flexion-type injury is similar to the injuries resulting from spearing, but less force is required to produce a flexion type of injury. The neck cannot protect itself in this hyperflexed position because the paravertebral muscles have lost their mechanical advantage in extending the neck. They now must exert their pull along the convexity of the arc, causing a compressive-type action, rather than an extension of the neck.

Stretching injuries result when blows from below strike the head in such a way that it is initially lifted up from the neck, thereby straining the ligaments that protect the intervertebral joints. If the force strikes the occiput of the head, in addition to stretching the neck, the head is forced into hyperflexion at the pivotal point in the center of the body of the vertebra. Great tensile strength of ligaments between the spinous processes, the *ligamentum flavum*, and the ligaments and capsules of the faceted joints is necessary in order to protect against bilateral locking of the facets as the posterior elements are pulled apart. If sufficient stretch occurs, the inferior articular facet of the vertebra above is lifted up and over the triangularly shaped superior facet of the vertebra below (Fig. 6-8). In the absence of rotation, this locking of facets occurs bilaterally. Since complete dislocation does not occur in such a situation, the subluxation may reduce spontaneously after impact, and only a chip fracture of the anterior-superior border of the vertebra will be demonstrated radiographically. The interspinous ligaments are usually not torn unless rotation occurs. If there is rotation, the result will be a unilateral facet dislocation. An example of a stretch injury occurs in boxing when a blow strikes under the chin. In this situation, the head is driven upward and backward causing a posterior dislocation, usually of C_5 and C_6. Although this injury is not likely to cause fracture, the dislocation can injure the spinal cord.

Hyperextension may be compressive or disruptive depending upon the direction of the blow. When the blow strikes the front of the head, the neck is forced through the stress and trauma ranges of motion, including translational and hyperextension. The anterior longitudinal ligament resists this motion, but the posterior bony arch is highly stressed at C_1. The lower spine is forced into extreme hyperextension. This situation would result from a blow of great magnitude, where the increased compressive force is expended on the posterior articular processes, spinous processes, laminae, and pedicles, forcing the vertebral body anteriorly. An intact anterior longitudinal ligament may cause this dislocation to reduce spontaneously.

Rotation injuries of the cervical spine are usually associated with other motion injuries, particularly with lateral flexion injuries. Lateral flexion injuries result from blows to the lateral aspect of the head or neck. In such injuries a lateral wedge compression of the vertebral body in the mid-cervical spine and a fracture of the transverse process occurs. If the force of the blow is sufficient, nerve roots may be avulsed with associated fractures.

In football, a blow delivered to the back of the ball player will suddenly propel his body forward, while his inert head, with its relaxed neck muscles, maintains its original position. This causes extreme hyperextension of the neck, followed by a precipitous pitch of the head forward into extreme

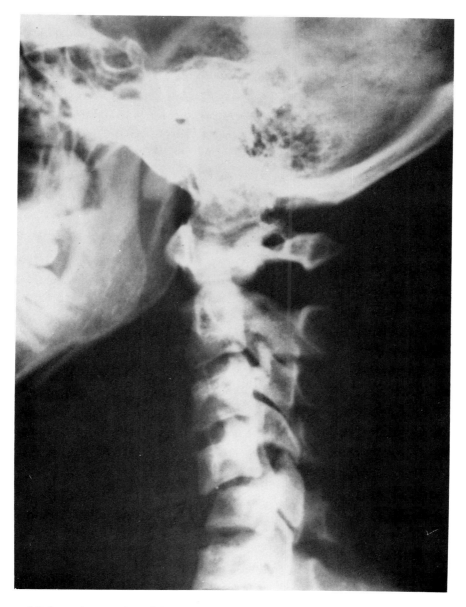

Figure 6-8. Lateral x-ray view of the cervical spine showing forward displacement of C_4 on C_5 as the superior facet of C_4 mounts the inferior facet of C_5.

flexion. This situation is referred to as whiplash.[7,19] The same mechanism occurs when the body is struck from the front. In this case the head would be whipped forward and the neck would be acutely flexed, followed by a spontaneous extensor recoil. The extreme mobility of the cervical spine often causes some injury to the muscle fibrils, with very little evidence of edema or hemorrhage. When a severe, unanticipated blow occurs, the neck travels beyond its normal range of motion into the stress and trauma range. The result is injury of connective tissue, tendons, ligaments, and articular capsules. Subluxation or dislocation of the joint then becomes inevitable. Although the chest may limit the downward motion of the chin during less severe impacts (in fact, during severe blows), once the chin strikes the chest rotation begins, causing the articular facets to be disrupted by the stretching of the capsules and ligaments surrounding these joints.

Brain Injuries

A linear skull fracture is not an indication of brain damage, but it does mean that the head has received a significant blow. Indentation of the skull rarely causes injury to the underlying brain, although occasionally a mild bruising of the brain occurs, and depressed skull fracture can cause a localized contusion or even a laceration of the brain substance. The significance of localized brain injury depends upon the area of the brain involved and, more importantly, upon any subsequent increase in intercranial pressure resulting from hemorrhage or swelling. Just as skull fractures can occur without brain injury, in contact sports brain injuries more commonly occur in the absence of skull fracture. These injuries are classified as accelerative or decelerative injuries and are due to sudden changes in motion of the head. Because the human brain is not as compact a structure as the brain of lower animals,[9] it is more easily injured as the result of sudden changes of motion. When the knee of an opponent strikes the head of a player, for example, a sudden change in motion occurs. This change may be in the form of a sudden reversal of the direction of motion of the player's head, a sudden cessation of motion, or a sudden commencement of movement. Any of these changes in skull motion occur prior to brain movement. This delay in brain movement can be compared to the delay in head movement in whiplash injury. In this situation, the body experiences a sudden change of motion as a result of impact, while the head lags behind.

The direction of a blow and the point of its impingement on the head determine the direction of skull motion. During translational motion, the head receives linear acceleration and rotational motion, causing angular acceleration. This may result in a shearing injury at the base of the brain as the irregular surface of the floor of the skull is put into motion. There is less likelihood of injury from motion over the smooth skull vault. Lesser degrees of motion, on the other hand, occur in the frontal and temporal lobes, which are confined in the more rigid anterior and middle fossae, and injury is more likely to occur here than in the parietal and occipital lobes, which are free to glide to absorb energy in their less restricted dural compartments. Sudden rotation of the skull may result in the tearing of blood vessels between the brain and the large venous sinuses. This venous bleeding increases intracranial pressure as a subdural hematoma develops.

Cervical Cord Injuries

The cervical cord occupies about one-half of the circumference of the bony cervical canal. It is injured when this protective housing is damaged, either by fracture of the bony parts or by dislocation of the intervertebral joints. The spinal cord, unlike peripheral nerves, is unable to repair itself once it has been damaged. Fortunately, less than one-half of the injuries of the cervical spine involving fractures or dislocations are associated with spinal cord damage.[10] Rotation of the cervical spine combined with either flexion or extension is necessary to produce a cervical dislocation and possible cord damage.

Peripheral Nerve Injuries

Brachial plexus injuries commonly occur in football and are referred to as burners or nerve pinches.[15,18] Forced lateral flexion of the neck is the mechanism of injury of these peripheral nerves. Two mechanisms are responsible for these injuries: (1) stretching of nerves on the side of the convexity of the lateral cervical spine flexion and (2) pinching of the nerves on the side of the concavity of the lateral flexion. Nerve stretch, especially of those components of the brachial plexus formed from the upper trunk, occurs when the interval between the intervertebral foramen and termination of the nerve is increased, as occurs when the head is forced into extreme lateral flexion and axial rotation and the shoulder is depressed. When an athlete assumes the blocking stance, his upper arms are brought away from his body and his fists are pressed against his chest. This increases the interval of the span of the axillary nerve as it travels posteriorly around the neck of the humerus to reach the deltoid muscle and overlying skin. The combination of all three conditions (i.e. forced lateral flexion of the neck, depression of the shoulder, and the blocking stance) can cause a stretching injury of the branches of the brachial plexus, especially of the axillary nerve on the side of the blow. Axillary nerve injury occurs more commonly in certain body builds, such as in the athlete with a long, thin neck with poorly developed musculature to offer resistance to lateral flexion. Furthermore, despite the fact that football players specifically develop massive neck muscles in order to strengthen their necks, these players frequently suffer recurrent brachial plexus stretch injuries. A possible explanation for this occurrence is that these peripheral nerves become entrapped in these overdeveloped muscles, particularly in the cleft between the anterior and medial scalene muscles (Fig. 6-9).

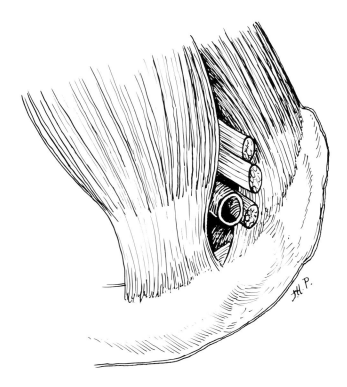

Figure 6-9. Hypertrophied scalene anterior and medius muscles inserting on the first rib could be an explanation for a brachial plexus pinch as these nerves escape in the cleft between these muscles.

Pinching of the components of the brachial plexus is more likely to occur on the side of the concavity of the lateral flexion at the point opposite the side of the blow. As the head is moved into extreme lateral flexion, axial rotation simultaneously occurs, causing the chin to rotate toward the side of the concavity. This combination narrows the intervertebral foramen, encroaching upon the nerve root and dural sleeve on the side opposite the blow.[3] Repeated trauma at the intervertebral foramen causes scarring and arthritic changes, further narrowing this aperture and increasing the irritation to the nerve root. In one instance, a heavily muscled guard suffered repeated trauma to the C_6 nerve root, resulting in atrophy and complete loss of strength in the triceps muscle. The nerve root was surgically explored for a probable disc injury; however, scarring and arthritic changes at the C_6 level were discovered to be responsible for this nerve injury.

MECHANISMS OF PROTECTION

The safest position for the head and neck with respect to impacts on the football field is in a neutral position, where the neck is held in a slight extension. With the head in this position, the player can see his opponent and is able to avert a direct hit to the axis of his spine. In addition, he can temporarily reduce the momentum of his opponent by calculated muscular resistance at the instant of impact, which prolongs impact time and permits pre-programmed muscular responses to become operative to further attenuate the blow, while the neck is moving within its normal range of motion.[6,8,11] As the stress range is reached, resistance is increased as the strong anterior and posterior longitudinal ligaments become taut and as the articular facets settle into their compressed position. Pre-programmed muscle response absorbs some of the energy of the blow by creating resistance during the time the head is traveling through its normal range of motion and by supporting the stopping action of the ligaments at the extremes of the range of motion. The muscles also function to prevent normal rotation of the cervical spine when this motion, coupled with flexion, could injure the interspinous ligaments and allow a unilateral facet dislocation. The important anterior and posterior longitudinal ligaments are also protected in forced extension when muscles act to prevent rotation of the cervical spine.

When a player is alert, he does not employ maximum resistance indiscriminately;[13] rather, he allows his controlled neuromuscular system to provide intermittent resistance in order to brake the momentum of his opponent over a longer period of time. When a player is in position to see an oncoming blow, he can make adjustments to vary his resistance, and he can even convert a direct hit into a blow that glances off his helmet. In such a situation the shoulder bears a large part of the intensity of the blow. The point to be stressed is that if a player resists to his maximum, he risks injury. The decision to offer calculated resistance insures that structural failure will not occur, and the player's neuromuscular system can respond as needed to support the function of ligaments and bones. This plan of response is equally as effective in stopping an opponent and markedly decreases the potential for injury. It must be noted that injury can occur even when the head and neck are in the optimum position at impact, especially in the case of a hyperextension compressive force of increased magnitude on a player with a long, thin, poorly developed neck.

SUMMARY

We can clearly see, therefore, that the high-intensity impacts that occur on the football field can have devastating effects upon the heads and necks of players in the game. Injuries that may even result in permanent disability can result when the athlete is reckless and offers too much resistance very rapidly. Injuries can also occur when very little resistance is offered and the head and neck are driven beyond their normal range of motion. An understanding of head and neck anatomy and physiology enables us to comprehend the mechanisms of these injuries. The ultimate protection from such injuries must come from the athlete himself, however, since even the most advanced helmet cannot provide complete protection. Through proper positioning combined with discriminate resistance, a player can decrease his injury potential without compromising his performance.

REFERENCES

1. Angel, R. W.: Antagonist muscle activity during rapid arm movements: central versus proprioceptive influences. *J Neurol Neurosurg & Psych, 40*:683, 1977.

2. Basmajian, J. U.: *Grant's Method of Anatomy*, 8th Ed. Baltimore, Williams & Wilkins, 1971, p. 577.

3. Cailliet, R.: The diagnosis of neck and arm pain by examination. *Ill Med J, 133*:277, 1968.

4. Carlsoo, S., and Johanson, O.: Stabilization of and load on the elbow joint in some protective movements. *Acta Anat, 48*:224, 1962.

5. Denny-Brown, D. E., and Russell, W. R.: Experimental cerebral concussion. *Brain, 64*:93, 1941.

6. Evarts, E. V., and Granit, R.: Relations of reflexes and intended movements. *Prog Brain Res, 44*:1, 1976.

7. Gehweiler, J. A., Jr., Osborne, R. L., Jr., and Becker, R. F.: *The Radiology of Vertebral Trauma*. Philadelphia, Saunders, 1980, p. 93.

8. Greenwood, R., and Anthony, P. H.: Landing from an unexpected fall and a voluntary step. *Brain, 99*:375, 1976.

9. Hirsch, A. E., Ommaya, A. K., and Malone, R. M.: Tolerance of subhuman primate brain to cerebral concussion. *Naval Ship Research and Developments Center Report*, Department of the Navy 1968, p. 2876.

10. Key, J. A., and Conwell, H. E.: *Management of Fractures, Dislocations, and Sprains*, 4th Ed. St. Louis, Mosby, 1946, p. 343.

11. Laursen, A. M., Dyhre-Paulsen, P., Djørup, A., and Johnsen, H.: Programmed pattern of muscular activity in monkeys landing from a leap. *Acta Physiol Scand, 102*:492, 1978.

12. Mertz, H. J., and Patrick, L. M.: Strength of response of the human neck. *SAE Transactions Paper]710855, 1971, p. 2903.*

13. Reid, S. E., Epstein, H. M., Louis, M. W., and Reid, S. E., Jr.: Physiologic response to impact. *J Trauma, 16*:150, 1975.

14. Roaf, R. A.: A study of the mechanics of spine injuries. *J Bone & Joint Surg, 42B*:810, 1960.

15. Robertson, W. C., Eichman, P. L., and Clancy, W. G.: Upper trunk brachial plexopathy in football players. *JAMA, 241*:1480, 1979.

16. Schneider, R. C.: *Head and Neck Injuries in Football Mechanism, Treatment and Prevention*. Baltimore, Williams & Wilkins, 1973, p. 17.

17. Schneider, R. C., and Kahn, E. A.: Chronic neurologic sequelae of acute trauma to the spine and spinal cord. Part I. The significance of acute flexion or tear drop fracture dislocation of cervical spine. *J Bone & Joint Surg, 38A*:985, 1956.

18. Turek, S. L.: *Orthopedics Principles and Application*. Philadelphia, Lippincott, 1977, p. 493.

19. Verriest, J. P., Martin, F., and Viviani, P.: Changes in the dynamic behavior of the baboon's head and neck system subjected to a frontal deceleration (-GX). *Proceedings of the Second International Conference Biomechanics of Serious Trauma*. Birmingham, England, Sept. 1975, p. 207.

20. White, A. A., III, and Panjabi, M. M.: *Clinical Biomechanics of the Spine*. Philadelphia, Lippincott, 1978, p. 21.

21. White, A. A., III, and Panjabi, M. M.: *Clinical Biomechanics of the Spine*. Philadelphia, Lippincott, 1978, pp. 71, 84.

Chapter 7

THE PHYSIOLOGIC RESPONSE OF MAN TO IMPACT

When an individual perceives himself to be in a potentially injurious situation (for the purpose of our discussion an impact of some type), all of his body systems prepare to respond. Stress is the trigger that sets the physiologic response into motion. In order to understand this response, which has been referred to by Selye as the general adaptation syndrome and termed alarm reaction by Cannon and de la Pax, it will be helpful to break down the reaction into its components, beginning with the response of the autonomic nervous system.[15]

AUTONOMIC NERVOUS SYSTEM RESPONSE

The autonomic or involuntary nervous system consists of two divisions: the sympathetic nervous system, which performs an excitatory function, and the parasympathetic nervous system, which performs an inhibitory function. The two systems thus function in opposition to one another, and each balances the actions of the other. For example, while the activity of the sympathetic nervous system causes an increase in the heart rate, the parasympathetic nervous system acts to slow this rate. The sympathetic nervous system is composed of fibers originating in each of the thoracolumbar segments of the spinal cord. Impulses to visceral organs are sent over motor pathways to the blood vessels, heart, lungs, endocrine glands, and sweat glands. Impulses are also sent over motor pathways via peripheral nerves to the skeletal muscles. The parasympathetic nervous system is composed of fibers originating in the cranial and sacral segments of the spinal cord, and its contribution to the physiologic response to impact is limited to its action on the heart and, possibly, the eye. As such, the activity of the autonomic nervous system tends to support the function of the central nervous system. It is the hypothalamus, located at the base of the brain, that is the center for regulation of the autonomic system, and it is this center that controls the body's reaction to stress.

102

ENDOCRINE SYSTEM RESPONSE

The endocrine system plays a significant role in the body's total physiologic response to impact. It consists of ductless glands that produce hormones and which are then carried by the bloodstream to their target organs. The endocrine glands involved in this response include the pituitary gland, or the hypophysis, and the adrenal glands. The pituitary lies under and is controlled by the brain. It coordinates and controls the actions of the other endocrine glands through the production of hormones. An adrenal gland, consisting of an outer cortex and an inner medulla, sits on the upper pole of each kidney. The cortex, when stimulated, increases the blood level of cortisone, setting the stage for action, with the highest levels being released during anxiety and very severe trauma. The liberation of catecholamines, called norepinephrine and epinephrine, by the medulla increases both the heart rate and the cardiac output. In addition, as vasoconstriction increases peripheral resistance, blood pressure rises and blood is shunted from inactive visceral organs, such as the spleen, and discharged into the general circulation. In emergency situations the sympathetic nervous system and the adrenal medulla function as a unit referred to as the sympathoadrenal system. When an individual is stressed or angered, this system coordinates the fight and flight responses.

NEUROMUSCULAR SYSTEM RESPONSE

The reaction of the neuromuscular system is the most obvious of the body's physiologic responses to impact. This system is comprised of skeletal muscles and peripheral nerves. Smooth locomotion is accomplished by muscles working in pairs: when one muscle, the agonist, contracts, its mate, the antagonist, relaxes. Muscles are made up of bundles of fibers, with each fiber a single cell. The characteristics of muscle depend upon its function, and it is the skeletal muscle only that concerns us here. Skeletal muscle varies in structural characteristics in order that it can most effectively respond to a variety of stimuli. For example, muscle fibers may be arranged in a somewhat oblique direction to the long axis of the muscle pull, in order to perform small, powerful movements. The fibers may also be arranged parallel to the long axis of the muscle, which means that they can shorten over a greater distance and move more rapidly over smaller distances. In addition to the differences in arrangement of muscle fibers, there are variances in their characteristics. The large, pale muscle fibers have a poor blood supply; they are easily fatigued and rarely used. When they are stimulated, however, rapid, powerful contractions occur. These fibers are innervated by large motor neurons, each supplying over one thousand pale muscle fibers. The muscle fibers involved in sustained contractions are red in color due to an increased blood supply that provides the fibers with nutrients and removes waste products that cause fatigue. These fibers are innervated by smaller motor neurons which supply fewer fibers. All muscles contain a muscle sheath (sarcolemma) and fibrous and elastic tissue.

The functional unit of the muscle is the motor unit consisting of one motor neuron and all the individual muscle fibers supplied by this nerve. Each muscle contains a variable number of these motor units. Intermixed among the muscle fibers of each motor unit are specialized receptors called muscle spindles. The spindles are stimulated when a muscle is stretched and impulses are carried over a segmental circuit or reflex arc to the spinal cord, across a single bridge or synapse, and are returned to the muscle for activation. This is the simple stretch reflex. It is interesting to note that in the extensor muscles of the neck, an unusually high spindle density is found.[11] This indicates that these muscles are particularly sensitive to stretch, affording increased protection from flexion injury to the cervical spine. The segmental circuits automatically regulate the length and tension of muscle in response to the mechanical input. They are controlled by signals received from higher centers of the central nervous system. A feedback control system regulates the action of these reflex responses by adjusting for any disturbances that may occur locally.[6]

REACTION TIME

The reaction time for a muscle to respond to stretch is the time from the commencement of stimulation of its spindles to the time of maximum contraction of muscle.[14] This time is divided into: (1) reflex time, or the total latent period, which extends from the time of stimulation of the receptor to the beginning of muscle activity elicited at the onset of the EMG; and (2) the contraction time, beginning at the onset of EMG activity to the maximum contraction of the muscle, which is noted at the peak of EMG activity. The reaction time of a reflex has been demonstrated experimentally to last as long as 120 milliseconds.

The type of stimulus directly affects the muscle reaction time. Auditory stimuli, for example, produce the slowest responses; visual stimuli produce faster reactions than auditory stimuli. It is the kinesthetic stimuli, however, that occur when a tendon is tapped, such as in a knee jerk, which have the fastest reaction time, measuring approximately sixty milliseconds.

The tone of the muscle immediately prior to stimulation of its spindles and before muscle contraction also influences reaction time. Muscle tone is defined as a state of involuntary, active tension, varying in intensity depending on the different actions that either inhibit or enforce it. It is tone that is responsible for the certain amount of tautness present even when muscles are at rest. If a muscle is slightly slack when stretched, the slack must first be taken up before the spindle receptors can be stimulated. Within a few milliseconds, the active state of the muscle leads to maximum tension, but this maximum tension can be maintained only for several milliseconds, after which it begins to deteriorate slowly to its resting tension. This takes place long before the stretch signal can traverse its reflex arc to cause contraction of the muscle. If muscle contraction reaches its peak EMG activity during maximum contraction of the active state, however, this maximum tension can be maintained. The amount of muscle tension during a panic or emergency situation is greater than it would be in a relaxed situation—sometimes amazingly greater. For example, a man who sees a child pinned under an automobile would be able, in this emergency situation, to raise the car up without assistance and rescue the child, a feat he would find impossible to duplicate later in a relaxed situation, even with the aid of two other men!

The speed of voluntary contraction is not limited by the mechanical properties of muscle fibers. If this were the case, large amplitude contractions required for greater forces could never be performed as rapidly as the small amplitude contractions required for lesser forces. The neuromechanism for increasing the speed and tension of muscle contraction at lesser force consists of the recruitment of additional motor units. At greater forces the primary mechanism for increasing the speed of tension is an increase in the firing rate to as much as 30 to 50 pulses per second from the normal 3 to 5 pulses per second. This is accomplished by repetitive stimulation of the sympathetic fibers, which increases the afferent discharge from the muscle spindles. Additional motor units are also recruited for increased strength.

In 1959, Miwa[12] stated that ligaments play a much greater part in resisting forces than is generally thought and that, insofar as distractive forces across the joint are concerned, muscles play a secondary role. This statement, however, is inconsistent with the fact that an unexpected blow to the head causes a whiplash injury, whereas injury rarely occurs when an individual is prepared to receive a blow. Reflex action alone has been demonstrated to be too slow and too weak to react to any type of blow, and voluntary muscle reaction is reported to be even slower than reflex action. Therefore, if muscle reflexes and voluntary muscle response are too slow to provide the necessary resistance to impacts, and ligaments and bony structures are similarly inadequate, there must be some other mechanism to account for the fact that man can protect himself against these high-intensity impacts, and that mechanism is the pre-programmed response.

PRE-PROGRAMMED RESPONSE

A very important factor in determining the reaction time of a voluntary movement is the proposed response of an individual to a particular stimulus prior to his actually receiving that stimulus. Experiments with monkeys who were trained to respond in only one manner to a stimulus (in this case by stretching their muscles) revealed a latency period of only 30 to 40 milliseconds prior to the onset of contraction.[3] When the monkeys were taught two responses to a given stimulus, this latency period doubled.[5] Experiments involving humans yielded similar results.[2] The fastest human reaction times occurred when the subject was fully aware of the direction of the impending disturbance and knew precisely how to react. Conversely, if both the direction of the impending disturbance and the response were unknown, there was a significant increase in the latency response, adding from 10 to 50 milliseconds to the response time.[2] These experiments demonstrate the importance of cortical preparation in reaction times. Such cortical preparation provides easy access to higher centers and presets the spinal cord reflex activity to perform in an efficient and specific manner. This cortical preparation for a particular response to stimulation is referred to as a pre-programmed response.[2,4,7,9,10]

Available evidence emphasizes the importance of pre-programmed muscular contractions, which are types of stored motor patterns for rapid voluntary movements. These movements, although initiated voluntarily, are primarily carried out automatically unless they are interrupted by some unexpected load. Pre-programmed behavior during impact has been studied using a man falling forward to the ground.[1] Protective movements of his arms set in motion muscular responses to cushion the fall. If the elbow joints were completely extended, great resistance would be exerted by these rigid bony extremities as the body was brought to an abrupt stop. The protective mechanism learned in childhood caused his elbows to be slightly flexed so as to reduce the force of impact by carrying out the braking action over a longer period of time. About 200 milliseconds prior to the start of the braking period, the activity of the flexor muscles of the upper arm was found to be significantly greater than when the braking was over. During the actual period of braking, strong muscular activity was interrupted by one or two silent periods, indicating that intermittent resistance occurred. This was especially true of the extensors of the forearm, where the activity started either simultaneously with, immediately before, or immediately after the commencement of the fall. Both agonist and antagonist muscles were found to be active in regulating the resistance required to carry out the braking action.

The EMG activity of the gastrocnemius muscle has been recorded in hopping movements in humans.[9] The studies concluded that muscular deceleration associated with landing was a direct result of a pre-programmed pattern of muscular activity and was not due to reflex action. Other experiments involving men suspended in parachute harnesses and dropped from varying heights revealed a peak of EMG activity in the soleus muscle of the calf of the leg in anticipation of landing.[7] A period of decreasing activity was noted immediately prior to landing. During each of the four trials used in this experiment, the subjects were instructed to concentrate on the landing platform. It was observed that the maximum of the EMG peak was related to the timing of the landing, which remained the same regardless of different heights of the falls. These peaks of EMG activity were considered to be caused by the voluntary cushioning response in preparation for landing, indicating that if the subject knows the height of the fall, he will be able to control his landing through pre-programmed muscular activity. A poorly developed pre-programmed response can be the result of errors in judgment, but it can also result when too many co-contractions occur, that is, activities of muscles which are not essential to the specific response. The number of co-contractions in a particular response is some indication of the training expertise of a player.

Through habit and experience, therefore, voluntary movements become established and refined pre-programmed behavior. A continual drilling of athletes to perfect skilled movements results in the successful repression of undesirable contractions and delays of spindle readjustment. This results in the onset of pre-programmed muscular action at or even before the moment of impact, which offers a calculated degree of resistance in order to avoid injury at impact.[8] It also serves to prolong the stopping time, allowing muscle activity to further cushion the blow. During triggered reactions, defined as selected pre-programmed movements superimposed on the stretch reflex, the stretch reflex can be enhanced resulting in a large increase in muscle stiffness.[2] Without these triggered reactions, which cannot occur during an unexpected disturbance, the stretch reflex is too weak to produce an appreciable counterforce to the impact.

The quick movements required to avoid injury on the football field do not allow time for the extensive sensory feedback; certainly there is insufficient time for voluntary responses to totally unexpected blows. In order to avoid injury, therefore, the cerebral motor command must be prepared and adjusted according to the expected force requirement. Furthermore, it is essential that the player remain alert to his environment so that he can react to the earliest auditory and visual cues signaling an impending impact. The preprogrammed commands are then sent in final form to the segmental circuits and motor neurons before the impact is initiated.

This type of pre-programmed response was observed in an instrumented player undergoing test impacts.[13] In anticipation of the blow, the player was observed to lean in the direction of the source of the blow, tensing all of his muscles and bracing himself for impact. His pre-programming resulted in his attempt to "feel" for the blow rather than indiscriminately offering maximum resistance. If he determined that the magnitude of the impact would be so great that structural failure seemed likely, he "rolled with the punch" and avoided injury.

This background study of muscle response gives some indication of man's ability to respond to impacts. The trained athlete, with his well-developed muscles and skills acquired through repeated exposures to similar situations, has perfected his response to high-intensity impacts. He has been pre-programmed and meets each blow with a calculated amount of resistance, sufficient to absorb some of the energy of the blow, thereby prolonging the stopping time and preventing injury.

SUMMARY

The total physiologic response to the threat of potential injury is a combination of the individual reactions from all of the body's systems—in particular, the autonomic nervous system, the endocrine system, and the neuromuscular system. It is the stress that results from the threat of injury that initiates the physiologic response.

The reaction time required for an individual to respond to a particular threatening stimulus is determined by his awareness of the potential threat (for our purposes, an impact of some type) and, assuming this awareness, the availability of a pre-programmed response to this stimulus. The pre-programmed responses that we have discussed in this chapter are the stored motor patterns for rapid voluntary movements that have been developed as a result of repeated exposure to the same or very similar situations. Because these motor patterns have become almost automatic responses, particularly in the case of the well-trained athlete, the pre-programmed response can begin immediately upon or even before the moment of impact, thereby greatly reducing the possibility of injury. It is our hope that a better understanding of the total physiologic response and of the importance of pre-programmed responses will lead to new approaches to the problem of player protection in football.

REFERENCES

1. Carlsoo, S., and Johansson, O.: Stabilization of and load on the elbow joint in some protective movements. *Acta Anat, 48*:224, 1962.
2. Crago, P., Houk, J. C., and Hasan, Z.: *Regulatory actions of human stretch reflex. J Neurophysiol, 39*:925, 1975.
3. Evarts, E. V.: Motor cortex reflexes associated with learned movements. Science, *179*:501, 1973.
4. Evarts, E. V., and Granit, R.: Relations of reflexes and intended movements. *Prog Brain Res, 44*:1, 1976.
5. Evarts, E. V., and Tangi, J.: Reflex and intended responses in motor cortex pyramidal tract neurons of monkey. *J Neurophysiol, 39*:1069, 1976.
6. Granit, R.: Constant errors in the execution and appreciation of movement. *Brain, 95*:649, 1972.
7. Greenwood, R., and Anthony, P. H.: Landing from an unexpected fall and a voluntary step. *Brain, 99*:375, 1976.
8. Hagbarth, K. E., Wallin, G., and Lofstedt, L.: Muscle spindle activity in man during voluntary fast alternating movements. *J Neurol Neurosurg Psychol, 38*:625, 1975.
9. Jones, G. M., and Watt, D. G. D.: Observations on the control of stepping and hopping movements in man. *J Physiol, 219*:709, 1971.
10. Laursen, A. M., Dyhre-Paulsen, P., Djørup, A., and Jahnsen, H.: Programmed pattern of muscular activity in monkeys landing from a leap. *Acta Physiol Scand, 102*:492, 1978.
11. Marsden, D. C., Merton, P. A., and Morton, H. B.: Latency measurements compatible with a cortical pathway for the stretch reflex in man. *J Physiol (London), 230*:58, 1973.
12. Miwa, N., and Metoba, M.: Quoted by Basmajian, J. V. In *Muscles Alive,* 3rd ed. Baltimore, Williams & Wilkins, 1974, p. 172.
13. Reid, S. E., Epstein, H. M., Louis, M. W., and Reid, S. E., Jr.: Physiologic response to impact. *J Trauma, 15*:150, 1975.
14. Schneider, L. W., Foust, D. R., Bowman, B. M., Snyder, R. G., Chaffin, D. B., Abdelnour, T. A., and Baum, J. K.: Biochemical properties of the human neck in lateral flexion. *Proceedings of the 19th Stapp Car Crash Conference.* Warrendale, PA: Society of Automotive Engineers, 1975, p 455.
15. Selye, H.: *The Stress of Life.* New York, McGraw, 1956.

Chapter 8

NECK MUSCLE RESISTANCE TO
HEAD IMPACT: AN EXPERIMENTAL STUDY

INTRODUCTION

This chapter describes a model that we developed to analyze the motion resulting from impacts of low-level intensity to a head and neck system. Movement of the head was limited to the normal range of motion; within this range, all resistance to head movement is caused by soft tissue, primarily muscle.[5]

A review of the literature on neck muscle response to a whiplash kind of head motion revealed that experimental work included measurements of reflex time,[1] data concerning the time required to stop the head motion,[2] and information regarding neck muscle response to impact in both humans and monkeys.[3,4,6,7] Mechanical models, which were built from a spring mass system, with a sphere representing the head and a spring representing the neck, frequently were employed to study this type of muscle response. These mechanical models cannot, however, duplicate the response of a human subject, nor can they provide a numerical value to the resistance produced in each test utilizing the model.[8] These limitations can be overcome by building a model that simulates a time-controlled spring mass system, utilizing a network of analog and digital computers that can change resistance parameters continuously and which offer no resistance when the neck muscles fail to respond.

EXPERIMENT

The purpose of our experiment was twofold: (1) to develop an acceleration-time curve of the response of human subjects to an externally applied force to the head and (2) to record muscle activity using electromyography (EMG). The collected data was stored in a digital computer for later analysis and simulation by an analog computer. The information obtained was used to verify the model, to demonstrate the manner in which neck muscles build up resistance to head movement, and to point out the specific parameters that influence reaction time. The experiment involved only tugs in the

Reprinted by permission of Aviation, Space, and Environmental Medicine, 52(2): 78–84, 1981. Copyright © by Aerospace Medical Association, Washington, D.C.

voluntary range of motion so that the peak force was limited to 38 pounds (170 Newtons), the duration of the force no longer than 50 to 70 milliseconds, and the peak acceleration limited to three gravitational units (3 G's).

The subject, who was seated in a chair, experienced a precise, sudden backward pull of his head in the median sagittal plane, accomplished by means of a system of pulleys and a falling weight (Fig. 8-1). The magnitude of the tug was recorded by a force transducer placed between the subject's head and the pull rope. Two accelerometers were mounted on the subject's forehead, oriented in the median sagittal plane: one in the anterior-posterior (X) direction, the other in the inferior-superior (Z) direction. Muscle activity in the sternocleidomastoid muscle was recorded by EMG using surface electrodes. The measured signals were amplified by AC amplifiers and then converted to digital signals (12 bits), which were stored on floppy computer diskettes.

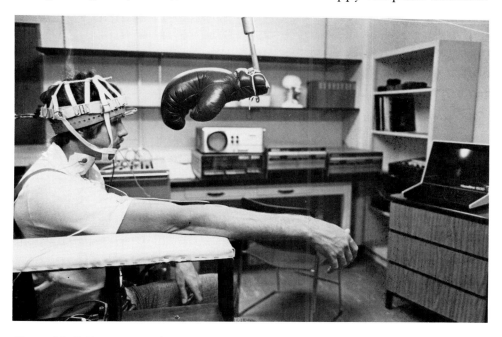

Figure 8-1. Pull rope secured to the head halter with force transducer EMG surface electrodes seen on right side of player's neck, accelerometers secured to player's forehead aligned in X axis and Z axis. Warning pendulum (boxing glove) arrives at head at instant of tug. Falling weight with warning lights on wall triggered by computer. Oscilloscope and computer in background. Amplifiers in wheeled cart at players left shoulder. Courtesy of Aviation, Space, and Environmental Medicine.

The experiment was controlled by the digital computer, which flashed instruction lights, released a warning pendulum, released a weight to fall after a pre-set delay, and which stored the information obtained from the

four data channels. The time interval between each operation was determined by the operator. The experiment was conducted in the following
combinations:

1. An unexpected tug on the head of a subject whose eyes and ears were
   covered.
2. An unexpected tug on a subject who was instructed how to react by
   lights that flashed at pre-set intervals prior to the tug.
3. An expected tug on a subject who saw the weight fall.
4. A release of a falling weight and the warning pendulum to allow the
   tug to occur at the instant the pendulum arrived at the subject's
   head.

The weights used varied from one to five pounds (0.5 to 2.5 kgs), with the
height of the fall ranging from 8 to 40 inches (20 to 100 cms).

MODEL THEORY

Our model was based on the following assumptions:

1. Motion of the head that occurs when an external force is applied
   along the X axis is a combination of two independent motions: (a) a
   linear motion of the head, which is very close in direction to the
   external force applied along the X axis; (b) a rotational motion of
   the head around its axis on the neck (AR axis, Fig. 8-2).
2. The magnitude of the tug on the head must be of low intensity in
   order to avoid the resistance that would occur at the extremes of the
   range of motion of the head and neck system. At these extremes, the
   limitation of motion at the bony joints would introduce a form of
   resistance that would interfere with our study of resistance produced
   by muscle and other soft tissue.
3. The head/neck responds as though it were a spring mass system.
   Oscillatory or vibratory motion is characteristic of a mass attached
   to a spring and occurs when the head receives a blow that causes
   neck muscles to be rapidly stretched. The velocity feedback from
   spindle receptors and certain mechanical properties of muscle cause
   a damping of this vibratory motion. Two modes of resistance are
   noted in the head/neck response. In the idle mode, the elasticity is
   equal to zero and the damping factor is less than 0.7 lb-sec/ft (10 N
   sec/m). In the resistance mode, elasticity is not equal to zero and the
   damping factor is somewhat larger than in an idle mode. When the
   subject resists, muscles are activated and the "spring" is in the
   resistance mode.
4. The elasticity and damping of the resistance mode are constant

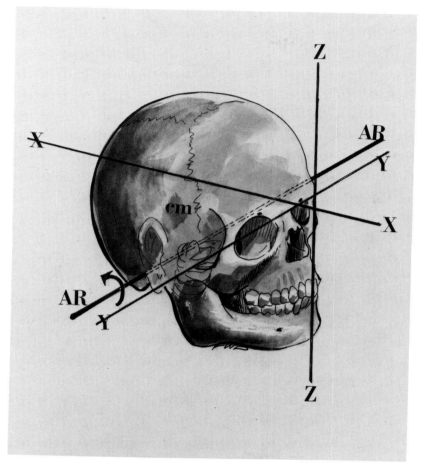

Figure 8-2. Three axes of the coordinate system (X,Y,Z) are depicted on a drawing of the human skull. The axes of rotation (AR) is shown at the atlanto-occipital joint. Courtesy of Aviation, Space, and Environmental Medicine.

throughout any single run, although different constants may be employed during different kinds of runs.

Assuming that head motion follows two separate directions (assumption 1), one could build a model to study each direction independently. The model would have to include a spring mass system (assumption 3), which would have the ability to vary resistance at any instant between an idle and resistance mode. In addition, the model would need to easily change its elasticity and damping factors in order to simulate the changes observed in the collected data of muscle response in the linear component of motion along the X axis. These requirements can all be achieved through the use of a network containing an analog computer connected to a digital computer. The analog computer simulates the spring mass system, having the capacity to insert the elasticity and damping parameters in a timely fashion with an "on" and "off" switch controlled by the digital computer. The analog computer behaves according to the formula for an oscillating mass, derived from Newton's Second Law, $F = ma$:

$$1.\ M\frac{d^2X}{dt^2} + [1 - Z(t)]\ B_1\frac{dX}{dt} + Z(t)\,B_2\frac{dX}{dt} + Z(t)\,KX = F(t)$$

where:

M = head mass
X = head displacement (in the X direction) as function of time
$\frac{d^2X}{Dt^2}$ = acceleration
B_1 = passive damping factor (no resistance to oscillation)
$\frac{dX}{dt}$ = velocity
B_2 = active damping factor (resistance to oscillation)
K = elasticity coefficient or spring stiffness
$F(t)$ = applied force as a function of time
$Z(t)$ = resistance exerted by the subject during his response to the tug
    = to one, if the muscles are activated
    = to zero, if muscles are inactive

The input of the analog computer ($F[t]$) is supplied by the digital computer and is the recorded force of the tug on a subject's head. The output of the analog computer, the head acceleration towards the negative X axis (d^2X/dt^2) is recorded and analyzed by the digital computer and then displayed for comparison with the head acceleration curve. In addition, the digital computer feeds the analog computer the function $Z(t)$ at the time pre-set by the operator.

As noted in the equation above, there are two variables that, together with the function $Z(t)$, determine the muscle resistance in the neck to decelerate head motion: (1) the elasticity coefficient (K) and (2) the active damping factor (B_2). The mass of the head (M) and the passive damping factor (B_1) are considered constant for any subject. During the single phase of resistance, when the subject begins to resist at some time after the tug starts, $Z(t)$ switches from zero to one and resistance continues until the head motion has ceased. In this case, the $Z(t)$ function is simply reduced to the reflex time of the subject.

The values of the damping factor and elasticity coefficient can be calculated approximately utilizing the acceleration curve of the muscle response and the force curve. These values are then fed into the model and provide the measure of resistance to the force variations stored in the digital computer at the exact time the digital computer has been instructed to open the

Z(t) switch. A model acceleration curve closely matching the variations in acceleration caused by muscle response to the tug is thereby produced. The calculated values of B_2 and K are corrected by trial and error to produce a model acceleration curve very similar to the muscle acceleration curve.

The process of determining these parameters can be demonstrated in Figure 8-3. (a) This is the resultant head acceleration curve along the X axis, and (b) this represents the force curve of the tug and is shown as a pulse with a duration of 70 milliseconds. Comparing these two curves, it appears that up to the break point at 90 milliseconds (see arrow), the acceleration curve is linearly related to the force curve. This suggests that during the tug the muscles are inactive (Z = 0). At the break point, a sudden change in the acceleration curve indicates that the subject has started to resist, and this resistance causes the deceleration of the head, as observed after the break point. This information leads to the conclusion that Z(t) is equal to zero up to the time of 90 milliseconds and that Z(t) is equal to 1 after 90 milliseconds. It can be seen that there is some deceleration between the time that the tug stops and the force curve returns to baseline, just before the break point occurs, indicating that the deceleration is due to the static damping factor. Also significant is the point where maximum deceleration occurs in the acceleration curve: at 120 milliseconds, the lowest dip in the curve, which indicates that the head has reached its maximum backward displacement and has started to return to its resting position. At this change in direction the head velocity must be zero; therefore, the damping term B_2 (dX/dt) at this point must also be zero. Since the tug now is also zero (F[t] = zero), then the only force remaining on the head is the elasticity force, and Equation 1 is reduced to:

$$2.\ K = \frac{-M\,(d^2X/d\,t^2)}{X}$$

Because the mass and acceleration of the head are known, X, the displacement of the head, can be found by two integrations of the acceleration data. We found that by using this method of calculation, elasticity could be determined with an error of 30 percent to 40 percent. The damping factor is more sensitive to measuring error and there is no simple way to compute it. The Z(t), K, and some reasonable value for the B_2 were fed into the model as approximate values. Then, by a trial-and-error method, the K and B_2 values were modified until an optimum curve was achieved. The model acceleration curve is illustrated in Figure 8-3c. The acceleration curve (Fig. 8-3a) and the model curve fit well up to the break point (arrow), at which time the subject begins to resist. A minor deviation of the curves occurs here because the resistance has been added abruptly in the model curve, whereas the resistance in the muscle curve actually builds gradually due to the delay in the contraction time of muscle. This deviation in the break point could be corrected, but it would complicate the equation. Its presence gives an accurate measurement of the contraction time of muscle (in this case, 35 milliseconds).

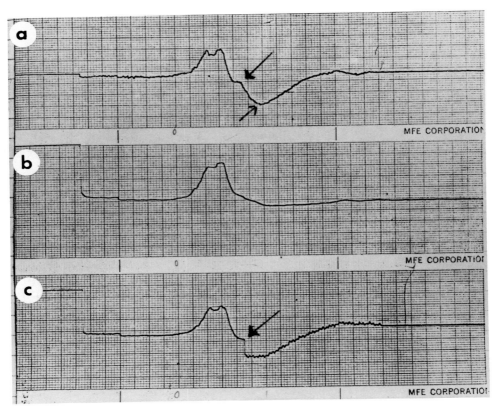

Figure 8-3. Comparison between (a) head acceleration curve and (b) force curve resulting from a tug of the head in a linear ($-X$ direction) when subject was instructed to resist at will and was unaware of what to expect. The two curves have a linear relationship up to the point of the arrow, when the subject started to resist and deceleration occurred. (c) The model acceration curve compares favorably with the upper graph (a). The model was run with a $Z(t)$ function changing abruptly from zero to 1 at the break point (arrow) at 9 ms. Muscle contraction time is measured from break point to point of upward-pointing arrow. ($K = 1500$ N/m and $B_2 = 15$ N s/m) Courtesy of Aviation, Space, and Environmental Medicine.

During some tugs, when the subject resisted as he desired, more than one phase of resistance occurred and more break points were seen in the acceleration curve (Fig. 8-4a). Additional data revealed the exact time at which the subject started to resist, for when resistance commenced, the muscle acceleration curve (Fig. 8-4a) failed to follow the force curve (Fig. 8-4b) and their linear relationship ceased. During some tugs, when the subject exerted a great deal of resistance, the elasticity (K) and even the active damping factor (B_2) could be calculated more accurately: K could be calculated from the time interval between two successive acceleration peaks; B_2 could be calculated using the ratio of the amplitude of these two peaks (Figs. 8-7b & 8-8b). Using the analog model for simulation was always more accurate than analytical calculation, but the latter was used to shorten the time necessary to reach the correct values, employing the trial-and-error method to arrive at a curve that would match the head acceleration curve.

RESULTS

Figures 8-3 through 8-8 represent the results. Figure 8-3 is the record of a run in which the subject was instructed to resist as desired. On the first run (Fig. 8-3c), the subject did not know what to expect; consequently, resistance was high: K = 100 lb/ft (1500 N/m), B_2 = 1 lb-sec/ft (15 N sec/m). The time required for the subject to initiate resistance was 90 milliseconds and muscle contraction time was 35 milliseconds. Similar results occurred in two successive runs in which the elasticity coefficient dropped to 50 lb/ft (750 N/m) and then to 43 lb/ft (650 N/m). This drop occurred once the subject realized that no real harm would result from the tug and relaxed. In these three runs the subject reacted just after the tug was over. When asked to resist as soon as possible but not prior to the tug, the subject would start to resist during the tug, with some responding after a time lapse of 25 milliseconds, very close to the muscle contraction time. Reflex time could be determined by measuring the latency between the start of the tug and the start of the EMG (Fig. 8-7a) or by observing the point at which the experimental acceleration curve and the force curve deviated from their linear relationships. When the subject was instructed to initiate resistance before the tug, the EMG started before the tug (Fig. 8-8a) and the values of K and B_2 were constant from the start to the end of the curve.

As we have mentioned, in some runs when the subject was instructed to resist as desired, multiple phases of resistance were noted. Figure 8-4 shows that the muscle acceleration curve (a) departed from the force curve (b) after 40 milliseconds, relaxed immediately after the tug was over, and then tensed again with another break point 100 milliseconds after the tug started. Further evidence that more than one phase of resistance occurred can be seen in Figure 8-5. Figure 8-5a shows the model acceleration curve that would occur if the subject resisted in only one phase, beginning 40 milliseconds after the tug started. Figure 8-5d illustrates the model acceleration assuming the subject resisted in one phase that began 100 milliseconds after the tug

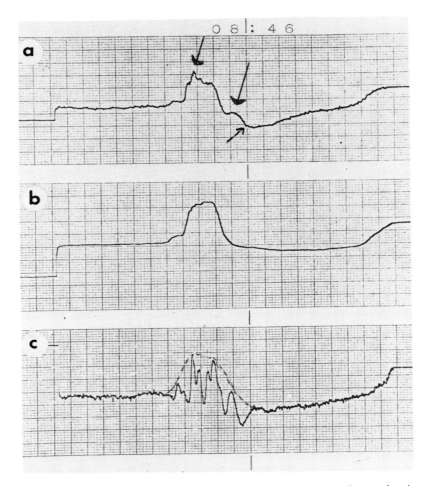

Figure 8-4. (a) Head acceleration in ($-$X) linear direction showing two phases of resistance (at arrows), (b) force curve, and (c) head acceleration in tangential (Z) direction. Dotted line joining peaks represents the envelope. Muscle contraction-time measured from second break point and upward-pointing arrow. Courtesy of Aviation, Space, and Environmental Medicine.

started. Finally, Figure 8-6a depicts the model deceleration curve assuming a double phase of resistance. There is no doubt that Figure 8-6a fits the muscle contraction curve more closely than the curves in Figures 8-5a or 8-5d, and that it could fit exactly by improving the model so that it had a gradual rather than a switching function for Z(t), as well as the ability to have different elasticity coefficients in each one of the resistive phases.

Tests were performed with three heavily muscled athletes who were instructed to respond in one of four ways:

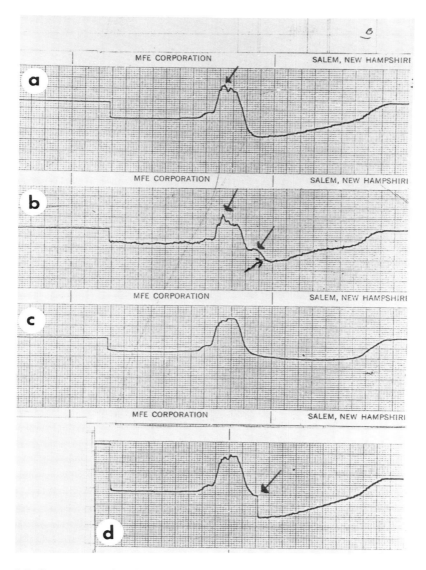

Figure 8-5. Same run as in Figure 8-4 showing the model curve with only one phase of resistance occurring at 15 ms (a) and a model curve with only one phase of resistance starting at 64 ms (d). The head acceleration curve (b) and the force curve (c), which is also shown in Figure 8-4, is included here for comparison with graphs a and d. Muscle contraction time measured between contiguous arrows in curve 5b is seen. Courtesy of Aviation, Space, and Environmental Medicine.

1. Not to resist at all
2. Resist as much as desired (Fig. 8-3)

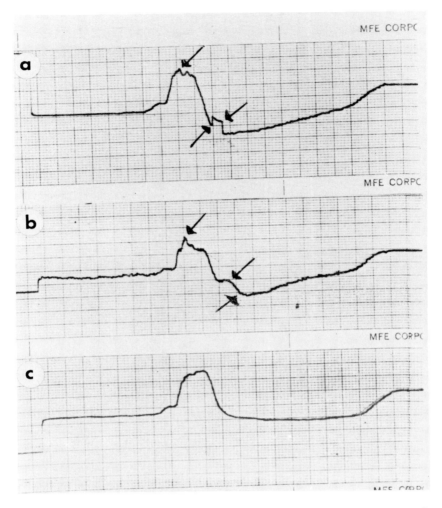

Figure 8-6. Same run as in Figure 8-4 with (a) the model curve showing resistance starting at 15 ms (arrow), stopping at 50 ms (arrow), and starting again at 64 ms (arrow). Lower curves are head acceleration (b) and force curves (c) for comparison. Courtesy of Aviation, Space, and Environmental Medicine.

 3. Resist as much as possible (Fig. 8-7)
 4. Resist as much as possible with a preload (Fig. 8-8)

Results were averaged and showed significant differences in the four types of responses. When the subject was instructed not to resist at all, K was less than 10 lb/ft (150 N/m), the range of error of the model. This tends to support the theory that during the idle mode, elasticity is negligible and that hard tissue (bone), which provides involuntary resistance, has no role in this range of impacts. When the subject was instructed to resist as much as desired after

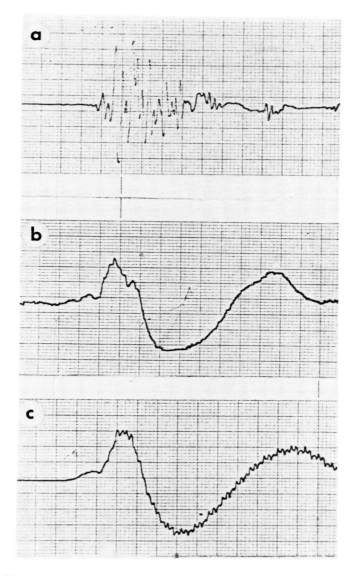

Figure 8-7. Subject instructed to resist as much as possible: (a) EMG; (b) head acceleration; and (c) model acceleration. (K = 2750 N/m, B_2 = 40 N s/m) Courtesy of Aviation, Space, and Environmental Medicine.

trial runs to acquaint him with the impact, resistance values ranged between K = 40 lb/ft (600 N/m) and 67 lb/ft (100 N/m), depending upon the subject, but the value of K for each subject was constant from test to test when each subject was given the same instructions on how to respond. When the subject was asked to resist as much as possible, the average value of K was 167 lb/ft

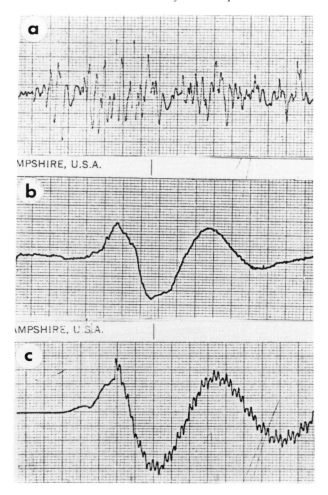

Figure 8-8. Subject instructed to resist as much as possible with a pre-load of 10 Kg in addition to tug: (a) EMG (muscle activity began before the tug started); (b) head acceleration ($-X$ direction); (c) model curve. (K = 7000 N/m, B_2 = 50 N s/m) Courtesy of Aviation, Space, and Environmental Medicine.

(2500 N/m) (Fig. 8-7) and the maximum was 183 lb/ft (2750 N/m). When asked to resist as much as possible with a preload, the resistance more than doubled to become K = 467 lb/ft (7000 N/m) (Fig. 8-7). While the K values increased more than 40 times between no resistance and maximum resistance with a preload, the increase in B_2 was far less striking. It was found that the mere presence or absence of resistance primarily accounted for the increase in the damping factor. Increases or decreases in resistance did not make a large difference in the damping factor.

In the section on model theory, two independent motions of the head were discussed and the component that occurs along the X axis was analyzed using an analog computer model. A similar model with minor changes can be designed to analyze the resultant motion along the Z axis in the inferior-superior direction. Figure 8-4c (lower graph) represents the acceleration curve of motion along the Z axis. The muscle contribution to this curve is shown by an envelope joining the peaks of the rapidly varying portions of this curve. This envelope is described in Equation 1, with mass being replaced by moment of inertia, displacement of the head replaced by angular head displacement, and torque substituted for force (F[t]). Within this envelope the real tangential acceleration is noted in the vicinity of the tug, but we still needed an explanation for the origin of these multiple peaks. We found that these peaks appeared even when the EMG was totally flat, which indicated that they were not caused by muscle contraction. If the peaks were caused by an external force, then values ten times greater than the actual force of the tug would be required. This indicates that abrupt stops occur successively during the deceleration of the head. Motion at each intervertebral joint is limited, each contributing to the total motion of the cervical spine. As each joint reaches its range of motion, a checking action occurs as the result of stretched intervertebral ligaments and bony stops of faceted joints. This could very well be the explanation for these multiple peaks of tangential acceleration.

DISCUSSION

A small group of eight subjects ranging in age from 18 to 23 years were selected from the various test trials. The group included one female and seven males of varying body builds. The elasticity coefficient of the woman was less than that of the men in all modes of resistance, with the most heavily muscled athlete having the largest elasticity coefficient. No significant differences in the reaction times were noted.

The tests revealed that K, B_2, and Z(t) were relatively constant, changing little during repeat runs. The only time that change did occur was when the subject was uncertain about the kind of impact he was to have or when he was instructed to alter his resistance. It was noted that the subject could fully control his resistance/non-resistance. When the subject resisted as desired, multiple phases of resistance were noted, indicating that intermittent muscle contractions were very likely due to local spindle stimulation. When he was instructed to resist as much as possible and as quickly as possible after the start of the tug, he reacted much earlier, sometimes after only 25 to 30 milliseconds, and a single phase of resistance was observed. This indicates that impulses from the brain prevented the local stretch reflex from becoming operative. It was surprising to note that during these small impact runs (weight drops between 1 and 5 pounds [0.5 and 2.5 kgs] and heights of drops from 8 to 40 inches [20 to 100 cms]), the elasticity of the neck muscles was the same regardless of the weight or height of the drop. This contradiction of the statement that the amount of resistance increases when the subject does not know what to expect might be explained by the fact that the subject was unconcerned about the differences in the tugs, knowing that none of the impacts would hurt him. We also found that the reflex and contraction times for the group were very close (about 25 to 30 milliseconds) and that the combinations of warning signals did not greatly influence the value of K, although they did somewhat improve reaction time. Warning was significant only when the subject was allowed to resist before the tug, and in these cases the reaction time was most efficient when the pendulum was used as the warning device. We are using the term efficient here to mean a measure of the subject's ability to postpone muscle activity until immediately prior to the onset of the tug and to regulate muscle activity during the tug.

It is clear from these experiments that neck muscles do provide resistance to head movement resulting from low-level impacts. We have observed that a subject is able to control the degree of the resistance of his neck muscles once he has become accustomed to the magnitude of the applied force. In this way he can resist in a safe, efficient manner. The main variables determining the resistance of a subject have been defined and their numerical values established. As a result of the experiments we have an accurate measurement of the contraction time of muscles under specific conditions. The ability to obtain this information is important when attempting to determine the effects of age, sex, physique, physical fitness, and training on the elasticity coefficient, the damping factor, reaction time, and contraction time. This information of the athlete's role in his own protection will, hopefully, add a new dimension to the means of avoiding injury to the head and neck.

SUMMARY

We have demonstrated that the exerted resistance under these conditions is a monotonic function of elasticity (K), and that this variable alone is sufficient to calculate the amount of a subject's resistance to an external force. Other variables are necessary only to resolve minor discrepancies between the muscle acceleration curve and the model curve of each particular impact. The resistance function (Z[t]) alone is sufficient for an examination of the parameters that influence the readiness or velocity of reaction of the subject. The small number of variables, combined with the ease in finding their numerical value, makes the model a powerful and useful tool for further research into the resistance exerted by neck muscles in head impacts.

REFERENCES

1. Foust, D. R., Chaffin, D. B., Snyder, R. G., and Baum, J. K.: Cervical range of motion and dynamic response and strength of cervical muscles. *Proceedings of the 17th Stapp Car Crash Conference.* Warrendale, PA: Society of Automotive Engineers, 1973, p. 285.
2. Hendler, E., O'Rourke, J., Schulman, M., Katzeff, M, Domzalski, L., and Rodgers, S.: Effect of head and body position and muscular tensing on response to impact. *Proceedings of the 18th Stapp Car Crash Conference.* Warrendale, PA: Society of Automotive Engineers, on response to impact. Paper No. 741184, 1974, p 303.
3. Huston, R. L., Huston, J. C., and Harlow, M. W.: Comprehensive, three-dimensional head-neck model for impact and high-acceleration studies. *Aviation Space Environ Med,* 49:205, 1978.
4. Mertz, H. J., and Patrick, L. M.: Strength and response of the human neck. *Proceedings of the 15th Staff Car Crash Conference.* Warrendale, PA: Society of Automotive Engineers, Paper No. 710855:207, 1971.
5. Reid, S. E., Raviv, G., and Reid, S. E., Jr.: Neck muscle resistance to head impact. *Aviation, Space and Environ Med,* 52:78, 1981.
6. Schneider, L. W., and Bowman, B. M.: Predication of head/neck response of selected military subjects to −GX acceleration. *Aviation Space Environ Med,* 49:211, 1978.
7. Schneider, L. W., Foust, D. R., Bowman, B. M., Snyder, R. G., Chaffin, D. B., Abdelnour, T. A., and Baum, J. K.: Biomedical properties of the human neck in lateral flexion. *Proceedings of the 19th Stapp Car Crash Conference.* Warrendale, PA: Society of Automotive Engineers. Paper No. 751156:455, 1975.
8. Verriest, J. P., Martin, F., and Viviani, P.: Changes in the dynamic behavior of the baboon's head and neck system subjected to a frontal deceleration (−GX) related to the action of cervical muscles. *Proc 2nd Int Conf Internat Res Comm on the Biokinetics of Impact.* Biomechanics of Serious Trauma, Birmingham, England, 1975, p. 207.

Chapter 9

IDENTIFICATION AND MANAGEMENT
OF HEAD INJURIES

We have included this chapter to provide information that will enable the medical team to recognize and identify head injuries that occur on the playing field in order that they may render appropriate first aid and determine the proper disposition of an injured athlete. Although head and neck injuries must be considered as a single entity, for the purpose of clarity they will be discussed in separate chapters.

AIRWAY

Ascertaining the condition of the airway of an unconscious, injured athlete is of paramount importance, since the unconscious player is unable to help himself and may have lost the gag and cough reflexes that normally cause any material collected in the nasopharynx to be forcibly ejected. An obstructed airway should be suspected when respirations are gasping, snoring, and slowed to less than eighteen per minute or when respirations become rapid and labored with periods when breathing stops momentarily and then resumes. In establishing a patent airway, however, it is critical to avoid doing further harm to a potentially serious neck injury. Since a fracture or dislocation of the cervical spine may have occurred, improper handling of the head and neck resulting from hasty and excited movements may expose the spinal cord to additional trauma. The mouth guard or any other foreign material, vomitus, or blood must be removed from the mouth to clear the airway and to avoid aspiration of this material into the lungs. The best position to allow such material to drain from the mouth is the semiprone position, where the injured player is turned halfway onto his stomach, neither completely over on his stomach nor directly on his side, bearing in mind that all movement of the unconscious athlete must be done only by the medical team (Fig. 9-1). In addition, the athlete's neck must be gently moved to a slightly extended position, which will allow material to drain freely from his mouth.[15] The strong anterior longitudinal ligament, which is rarely torn, will tend to splint the cervical spine when it is moved to this slightly extended position (Fig. 9-2). The injured athlete must be kept in this position, with his head and neck supported by sandbags or rolled towels, if it becomes necessary to transport him by litter to the hospital. His helmet should not be removed at this time, but the easily detached faceguard can be separated from the helmet by cutting the clamps that fasten it to the helmet. Removing the faceguard permits access to the face if further treatment of the airway is required.

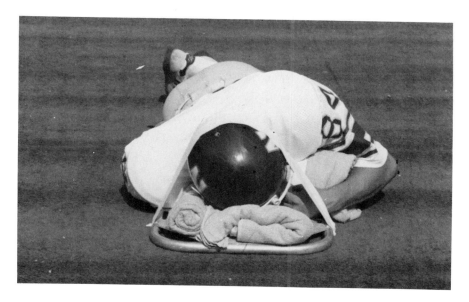

Figure 9-1. Semiprone position.

The relaxed muscles of the unconscious athlete will cause the lower jaw to fall open, with the tongue moving to the back of the throat and closing off the airway (Fig. 9-3a). This condition is sometimes referred to as a swallowed tongue and can be corrected by placing the fingers of each hand behind the angles of the mandible and pulling the relaxed, open lower jaw forward (Fig. 9-3b).

It is imperative that immediate attention be given to the condition of the airway in an unconscious, injured athlete because a cleared airway allows for the free exchange of air in the lungs, thereby preventing or minimizing brain damage that would occur if the delicate brain cells were deprived of adequate oxygen for a period of approximately five minutes. If necessary, an oral airway can be inserted in the unconscious athlete prior to transfer to the hospital (Fig. 9-4).

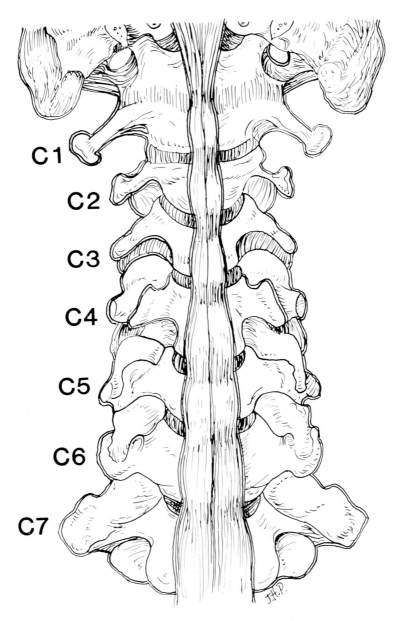

C1

C2

C3

C4

C5

C6

C7

Figure 9-2. Strong anterior longitudinal ligament.

a.

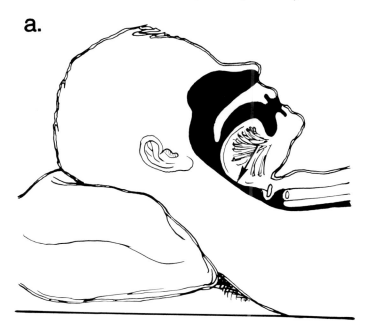

b.

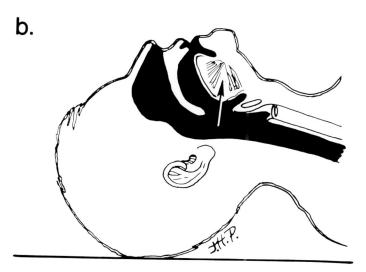

Figure 9-3. (a) In the unconscious athlete, the relaxed tongue drops back against the posterior pharyngeal wall obstructing the airway. This is the "swallowed tongue." (b) Extension of the neck opens the airway.

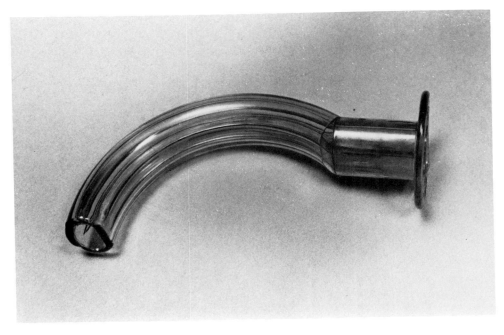

Figure 9-4. Oral airway.

SHOCK

The status of the circulatory system must be the next consideration of the medical team. Because shock is rarely the result of a head injury alone, it must be considered as part of the multiple injury complex. Additional injury sites may include fractures of long bones or hemorrhaging in the lungs or abdomen. A fast, thready pulse in the unconscious athlete, whose normal pulse rate is about 60 per minute, is the best indication of shock. In this situation, the athlete must be immediately removed from the field and transported to the hospital, with his blood pressure continually monitored in transit. In the absence of a pulse and respiration, cardiopulmonary resuscitation (CPR) must be instituted, requiring that the medical team have had training in CPR and be proficient in its administration.

HEAD INJURIES

Integument

The soft tissue of the head, including the scalp and the skin covering the face, has a very good blood supply and, as a result, bleeds quite freely when injured. Although such bleeding may appear excessive, it can be quite easily controlled by means of gentle pressure applied on top of a piece of sterile gauze. We know of one instance where the team physician was called to treat an athlete who had a bleeding laceration of the lip. The attendant was trying unsuccessfully to stop the bleeding by dropping adrenalin on the profusely bleeding wound. When a dry, sterile gauze was used to cover the wound and the athlete applied pressure to the cut, the bleeding stopped. After the bleeding has been controlled, and provided the laceration is not serious, it is perfectly safe to allow the player to continue in the game, since these injuries are considered to be clean/contaminated wounds for six hours. During this time period, such wounds can be closed in most cases by suture.

Nasal Injuries

Since the use of the face mask became popular, fractures of the nose and facial bones do not occur frequently in football, but they are relatively common in the sports of basketball, baseball, boxing, and ice hockey. A fracture of the nose, when seen early before soft tissue swelling occurs, can be easily detected by observation, and a deviated nasal septum caused by fracture should always be suspected when an athlete is unable to breath freely through both sides of his nose. Gross deviations of the nose to one side of the face may be corrected by applying gentle pressure to the nose, aligning it to the middle of the face. If further manipulation is necessary, the nose can be anesthetized with a topical application of cocaine applied with cotton applicators to the inside of each nostril. A blunt instrument may then be gently inserted into each nostril and the nose molded over the instrument with the fingers and thumb on the outside of the nose.

Nosebleeds are common in sports injuries, and the location of the bleeding point determines the method of treatment. A bleeding point in the anterior part of the nasal cavity can be easily controlled by pinching the nostrils together with the thumb and index finger. During this procedure the athlete should be in an upright position to reduce the congestion in the nose and to avoid blood running down into the nasopharynx. If pinching the nose is unsuccessful at stopping the bleeding, the nose can be gently packed with gauze moistened with adrenalin (1:1,000). In most instances, this should stop a mild hemorrhage. Any instrumentation of the nose must be performed under sterile conditions in order to avoid infection.

Facial Bone Injuries

Fractures of facial bones, particularly those overlying the paranasal sinuses, occur as a result of minimal force. They can often be diagnosed by simple palpation and comparing the two sides of the face. Fractures of the orbital rim surrounding the eyeball may result in double vision and occasionally cause an inequality of pupils. All fractures of the nose and facial bones should be x-rayed for confirmation.

Mouth Injuries

Injuries to the inside of the mouth are not common in football. Lacerations of the tongue result from a blow under the chin, which causes an athlete to bite his tongue. Since the tongue is primarily a muscle, it has a good supply of blood and will bleed freely. Very little treatment is required, however, except to control the hemorrhaging, and this can be done by placing some dry gauze against the wound. These wounds heal very readily and rarely require suturing. A white curd will appear at the site of the injury and is part of the normal healing process.

An injury to a tooth requires the care of a dentist. If the tooth is knocked out, it should be wrapped in sterile gauze and sent immediately with the injured player to the dentist. These teeth can often be restored to their original position if prompt dental care is initiated.

Fractures of the jaw are another common football-related injury. Such fractures can be identified from complaints of an uncomfortable, abnormal bite. These injuries should be confirmed by x-ray and treated by a plastic surgeon; an ear, nose, and throat specialist; or an oral surgeon.

Ear Injuries

When the ear is rolled against the head, bleeding may occur under the skin overlying the cartilage of the ear. This type of injury is most common in wrestling (Fig. 9-5). When the blood accumulates, it lifts the skin away from the normal contour of the ear cartilage, resulting in a potential cauliflower ear. The blood then clots and forms a scar under the skin overlying the ear, causing a permanent loss of the architecture of the external ear. If these injuries are neglected, plastic surgery will be required to remove the clots from the underlying cartilage and correct the deformity. Ideally, the ear will be treated the day after the injury. Under sterile conditions the blood will be aspirated with a fine gauge needle (25 g) and syringe, and a collodion cast will be applied to the injured ear.[20] The cast is formed by placing a thin layer of cotton over the ear and then applying flexible collodion to this cotton patch in multiple layers to form a thick, hard cast, with care taken to prevent the collodion from draining into the ear canal. The cast will hold the skin down over the contours of the cartilage and allow it to heal in its normal position without further treatment (Fig. 9-6). After the cast has been applied, it is imperative that there be no external pressure to the ear, such as wrapping an Ace bandage around the head. Not only is such additional pressure painful, it can result in necrosis of the ear cartilage with subsequent permanent deformity.

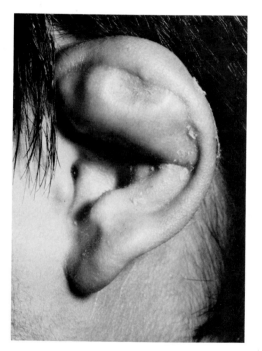 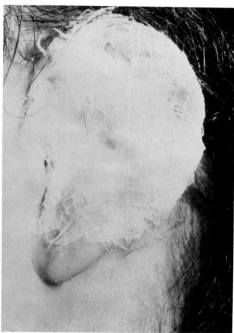

Figure 9-5. Shows the extent of bleeding under the skin covering the ear cartilage.

Figure 9-6. Collodium cast keeps gentle pressure over the convolutions of the ear cartilage.

Following this type of injury, the athlete is warned not to participate in the sport for a week in order to allow healing to occur. At the end of a week, the cast will separate from the ear and no further treatment is needed.

Eye Injuries

Serious injury to the eye is uncommon in sports, but minor injuries do occur.[1] The conjunctiva is a continuous, clear membrane that lines the undersurface of both eyelids and is reflected over the eyeball to form the conjunctival sac. Foreign bodies often lodge within this sac, causing considerable irritation and tearing of the eye. These foreign bodies can be removed with a moistened cotton applicator swabbed along the lower part of the sac. By applying pressure, the lower lid can be everted and the foreign body can be visualized by having the athlete move the eye in all directions. A foreign body lodged under the upper lid cannot be seen unless the eyelid is everted by having the athlete look down and then pulling the eyelashes of the lid down and away from the eyeball, then rolling the lid up over an applicator stick (Fig. 9-7). This exposes the conjunctiva, whereupon foreign bodies can be seen and easily removed. Following removal of a foreign body, the conjunctival sac must be irrigated with a boric acid solution to wash away any remaining irritants. Any foreign body lodged in the eyeball must be considered serious since it can injure the cornea, and referral to an ophthalmologist for its removal is indicated. A hemorrhage occurring under the conjunctiva may produce an angry-looking red eye, but, in the absence of visual loss, this is of no significance and will quickly resorb.

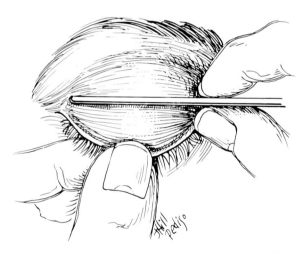

Figure 9-7. The method for turning the tarsal plate of the upper eyelid to check for foreign bodies under the upper lid.

After any eye injury, a player must be examined for evidence of more serious damage, and he must have his visual acuity checked to verify that he has good vision throughout his visual range. Any loss of vision must be investigated, with the retina observed with an ophthalmoscope for evidence of hemorrhage or of retinal detachment, which occurs rarely.[6] It must be remembered that loss of vision may be of a central origin, resulting from injury to the brain, or to some vascular change, such as the type of loss that occurs with a kinking of the vertebral artery at the base of the brain.

Skull Injuries

Skull fractures are uncommon in organized football games and occur infrequently in other sports where missiles are involved, such as baseball, track, or hockey. A skull fracture can rarely be diagnosed without the benefit of an x-ray examination, and even when a fracture is present, it is of no great concern for the medical team on the field, since it is principally an index of the severity of the blow to the head. Once any critical injuries have been given necessary attention, a radiographic examination of the skull is indicated.

Intracranial Injuries

The rigid skull protects the delicate nervous tissue of the brain, but brain injuries may still occur. When there is such an injury, the brain tissue swells due to edema or bleeding. Pressure results from this swelling, since the brain is expanding within the unyielding, closed compartment of the skull. The severity of the injury is determined by the degree of increased intracranial pressure. For example, the bleeding that results from injury to an artery results in brisk bleeding of high pressure and produces a rapid increase in intracranial pressure. On the other hand, the bleeding caused by a torn vein or blood sinus is under low pressure and symptoms develop gradually. There is a gradual onset of brain edema, and the resultant symptoms progress in a similarly slow manner; however, localized pressure in vital centers in the brain stem produces life-threatening symptoms early.[16]

Bleeding may occur in the absence of brain injury and may be of the following types:

1. Epidural or extradural, between the skull and dura mater. This bleeding is usually of arterial origin and results from a linear skull fracture across the middle meningeal groove in the temporal bone, which is located in front of the ear.[2,17]
2. Subdural, resulting from a tear of the major dural sinus or of the bridging veins between the brain and dura mater.
3. Injuries to the brain substance cause subarachnoid hemorrhage or intracerebral bleeding.

Brain injuries may be due to concussion, contusion, or lacerations. A concussion causes some loss of consciousness, with little, if any, gross brain injury, and it is likely to be temporary.[19] This deranged neural function usually lasts less than five minutes and is probably due to brain shock, which is similar to spinal cord shock that results in momentary paralysis of the extremities. A contusion is a bruising of a localized area of the brain with some associated bleeding. It is accompanied by a loss of consciousness that usually persists longer than five minutes.[5] Brain laceration is associated with intracranial bleeding and results in a prolonged period of unconsciousness. Intracranial bleeding occurs in 50 percent of patients who have experienced unconsciousness lasting approximately one hour or longer.

POST-CONCUSSION SYNDROME

Post-concussion syndrome occurs in an athlete who has developed an anxiety over his physical condition long after all neurologic findings have returned to normal.[7] This post-traumatic neurosis is characterized by complaints of persistent headaches, generalized weakness, giddiness, loss of initiative, and the inability to concentrate. In one instance an athlete who had recovered from a head injury continued to complain of prolonged headaches, which caused him great consternation and poor memory retention. After many conferences and examinations, the player was referred to a psychiatrist. Once he understood that his symptoms were psychosomatic in origin and not the result of residual brain injury, his symptoms ceased. It must be noted here that this syndrome is not always so easily remedied, but it is important to remember that following a brain injury, the athlete needs reassurance and positive input.

DRUG ABUSE

The athlete who takes drugs in the hopes that he will perform in a superhuman fashion needs to recognize that this strength is merely an illusion and that the drugs have produced a false sense of confidence. Phencyclidine hydrochloride, dubbed "PCP," "angel dust," "peace pill," "angel mist," "sheets," and "hog," produces agitation and excitement in small doses; in larger doses, stupor, coma, and death result.[3] Because these drug-induced symptoms mimic those found in head injuries, the athlete must be removed from the game and observed for evidence of serious intracranial injury. In one particular Tribune All-Star Game, an athlete came off the field appearing agitated and had a glassy-eyed stare. Although the player repeatedly denied that there was anything wrong with him, nonetheless he was benched. He later admitted to taking drugs.

REPEATED BLOWS TO THE HEAD

Most of the head injuries that occur in sports are regarded as essentially reversible in nature, without residual detectable brain damage. There is, however, developing evidence which suggests that repeated blows to the head may result in cumulative brain damage. In one experiment, Gronwall and Wrightson[8] tested a group of young, healthy, male adults, each of whom had two previous concussions. These subjects, when tested, were unable to process numerical information as rapidly as the control group composed of individuals who had a prior history of only a single head injury. The researchers also found that recovery was slower in the twice-concussed group, although in both groups the processing ability eventually returned to normal. Roberts[12] has also conducted clinical studies of brain damage resulting from boxing injuries in order to investigate the effects of repeated head blows. He, like Gronwall and Wrightson, concluded that repeated blows to the head may result in cumulative damage to the brain.

The Punch-Drunk State

The punch-drunk condition develops as a result of repeated head injuries, but it does not appear until several years after these injuries.[10] It is most common in boxers.[4] Symptoms of this condition are generally limited to the extremities. There may be a slight slapping of one foot when walking or the gait may be a bit unsteady. Slight mental confusion and a slowing of muscular action can also occur. Although symptoms may not always be progressive, muscular control in some individuals continues to deteriorate, leading to speech problems, hand tremors, and head nodding. Severe brain damage is demonstrated by a dragging of one or both legs, a staggering, propulsive gait, and a masked facial expression. The symptoms of tremors, dizziness, and deafness are followed by mental deterioration. Massive cortical scarring is found in the brains of those athletes suffering from this condition.[9]

In one study involving 1,200 boxing matches in which concussions occurred, boxers were neurologically compared with 1,000 non-boxers of similar age. The findings revealed that 9 percent of the boxers who received concussions later developed chronic boxer's encephalopathy.[18] Although proponents of boxing argue that the incidence of degenerative changes are no more common in boxers than in the general population and that this syndrome is found in athletes other than boxers, the evidence suggests otherwise. Corsellis[4] sent questionnaires to 165 British neurologists and requested their experiences with the punch-drunk condition either in boxers or other athletes. While only 22 cases were reported in non-boxers, there were 290 reports of the condition in boxers.

EXAMINATION FOR INTRACRANIAL HEAD INJURY

The unconscious athlete on the field must be examined in the position in which he is found and must not be moved until a thorough examination has been performed, since any loss of consciousness, even momentary, must be considered as serious. Haste is definitely not warranted during an on-field examination for a possible head injury. Periods of unconsciousness usually last less than a minute, and during this time the athlete should be observed for any random movements of his extremities or for any other injuries or abnormalities. After several seconds, the athlete usually recovers consciousness and is able to give an accurate description of his symptoms and the mechanism of injury.

The medical team must understand that an on-field diagnosis of the extent of a head injury is impossible. The primary function of the team is to see that no further injury occurs. Because the neurologic signs of a seriously injured player will change from minute to minute and from hour to hour, the medical team must maintain an accurate record of the initial findings to use later as a baseline guide. Periodic notations of changes in these signs must be entered into the record, and this record should accompany the patient to the hospital. Since most head injuries are diagnosed only after some time has elapsed, the physician at the hospital will have, immediately at hand to aid him in his diagnosis, a complete record of the length of unconsciousness and the sequence of the development of any neurologic deficits. The importance of these records cannot be overemphasized.

We will now discuss the neurological signs of intracranial injury in the order of their importance.

Level of Consciousness

The level of consciousness is the most important observation made by the medical team, and these observations must be extremely specific to be of value. Observations include:[14]

1. *State of Alertness.* The *slightest* change in mental acuity must be recorded. For example, are there symptoms of lethargy or drowsiness? Can the athlete be easily aroused from this lethargic state? Is he able to give intelligent responses to questions?
2. *Ability to Cooperate.* Is the athlete able to respond to commands, such as a request to move one extremity after the other, or to squeeze the hand of the examiner?
3. *Time Orientation.* Can the athlete tell the examiner the score of the game or the name of the opposing team? Even though the athlete may know where he is, he may have no concept of time.

4. *Place Orientation.* Disorientation to place is a sign of further clouding of consciousness. In this situation an athlete is unable to recognize familiar surroundings.

5. *People Orientation.* An athlete who fails to recognize his teammates or others familiar to him is clearly suffering the effects of impaired consciousness. Failure to respond to his own name demonstrates additional lethargy.

6. *Response to Painful or Noxious Stimuli.* Does the athlete draw back from the odor of ammonia spirits? When the thumb of an attendant is pressed against the bony ridge above the player's eyes, does he push the thumb away, does he make purposeless movements, or does he exhibit no response at all?

The variety in levels of consciousness can be demonstrated by the following three examples. The first example involves a quarterback who had been sacked and who left the field when the ball was turned over. Although this player showed no evidence of a head injury and no loss of consciousness, he was nevertheless unable to remember the score of the game or recall what had transpired in the previous three quarters. The second case concerned a middle guard who had received a head injury. He was knocked unconscious, but after a minute he came to and walked off the field. Once he returned to the bench, he demonstrated symptoms of amnesia: he did not know the score of the game, nor could he recognize his teammates. In addition, he repeatedly asked how he got hurt, but he was unable to retain this information when it was explained to him. He continued asking the same question throughout the remainder of the game. The third example involved a defensive tackle who had received a head injury in making a tackle and was unconscious for about a minute. After he had been brought off the field and into the dressing room, his total disorientation became obvious. He was unaware that he was playing in an out-of-town game, he had no recollection of his injury, nor could he remember the score of the game. Although he was a senior at Northwestern University, he could not recall ever having attended the school. The prolonged period of amnesia demonstrated by this player, in spite of a rather brief period of unconsciousness, indicated a more severe degree of head injury.

Eye Signs

The eye signs must be considered immediately after the level of consciousness has been determined in the evaluation of an athlete with a head injury. The iris is the color portion of the eye and is a reflex shutter mechanism controlled by the autonomic nervous system. The darkened aperture in the center of the iris is the pupil, and when the iris is stimulated by a bright light, the pupil constricts to pinpoint size; conversely, it enlarges in the absence of light. The equality in the size of the pupils of each eye, as well as their reaction to light, are an important observation in the diagnosis and localization of brain injury. Inequality of pupils is a more valuable localizing sign than is their reaction to light, but the latter finding must also be recorded. Even the subtle finding of a slight drooping of an upper eyelid, called ptosis, may be an indication of an impending problem. The pupils should always be examined early following a head injury because swelling and ecchymosis of eyelids are likely to occur in a very short time, making it impossible to open the eyelids, even when the fingers are used to pry the lids apart. A slight inequality of pupils may come and go, and this is usually an unimportant finding.

Inequality of pupils occurring early post-injury is frequently the result of a local eye injury. When this finding occurs later, however, the possibility of a brain stem injury must be considered. The finding of a unilateral dilatation or loss of the light reflex occurring some time after injury is usually the result of brain swelling or a hematoma formation under the dura mater. In 90 percent of the cases, the finding of inequality in pupil size indicates that the brain injury has occurred on the same side of the head as the dilated pupil.[22] A unilateral dilatation of the pupil with weakness or paralysis of muscles on the opposite side of the body also indicates brain injury. Dilatation of both pupils combined with a loss of the light reflex and with deteriorating levels of consciousness indicates serious brain injury. Bilaterally constricted pupils can occur as the result of diffuse brain damage caused by impairment of the sympathetic nervous system. Inequality of pupils with no other findings suggest the existence of a previous eye injury. Finally, bilaterally dilated pupils without evidence of brain injury may occur if an athlete is particularly anxious.

Following a head injury, the athlete must be checked for impairments of his visual acuity, of his fields of vision, and for double vision. Examination of the retina of the eye with an ophthalmoscope is not indicated early post-injury because brain swelling around the optic nerves occurs later. A detached retina can occur early, however, and if this condition is suspected, the retina must be examined immediately with an ophthalmoscope.

Although contact lenses are of great value to the athlete in sports such as tennis, handball, and racketball, players wearing contact lenses should also wear protective eyeguards to prevent injuries resulting from being struck in the eye by the ball.[21] Soft contact lenses seem to be better tolerated and are less likely to dislodge and pop out.

Reflex Signs

Once the eye signs have been evaluated in an athlete receiving a head injury, the medical team must turn its attention to the player's reflexes. Any involuntary movements, quivering, or spasticity of muscles must be recorded. In addition, the strength and range of motion of the extremities must also be noted; the responses on one side should be compared with the responses on the opposite side of the body. A determination of muscle strength is made by having the athlete squeeze the hands of the attendant. Despite the fact that these are gross tests, little other examination is required while the athlete is still on the field. Once the athlete has been removed from the field to the training room, then his reflexes should be thoroughly tested.

Superficial reflexes are those elicited by gently stroking the skin, usually with a blunt instrument. To elicit the abdominal reflex, the skin is stroked beginning at the navel, moving radially into the four abdominal quadrants. An intact superficial abdominal reflex is indicated by the movement of the navel toward the point of stimulation of the skin. The cremasteric reflex is elicited by stroking the inner aspect of the thigh and noting contractions of the cremasteric muscle as the testicle is drawn up in the scrotum.

Deep tendon reflex is elicited by smartly tapping the muscle near its attachment to the tendon, which should produce a tendon jerk. A biceps tendon is tested by tapping the tendon with a reflex hammer when the elbow is flexed to an almost 90-degree angle. A positive deep tendon reflex will cause the biceps muscle to twitch. The triceps reflex is elicited in a similar manner by tapping the muscle just above the elbow on the extensor aspect of the arm, causing a twitch of the triceps muscle. It is often impossible to see the action of the tendon reflex, but it can be felt if a finger is applied over the muscle. A knee jerk is elicited by tapping the tendon just below the kneecap when the knee is in a relaxed, right-angle position. This should produce a twitching of the quadriceps muscles in the front of the thigh.

A pathological reflex occurs when there has been an injury to the base of the brain. The Babinski reflex may be elicited by stroking the lateral aspect of the sole of the foot. In a normal reflex, the toes will curl in flexion, but in the pathological state, the great toe is extended and the four remaining toes may be extended into a fanned position.

Reflex changes are significant signs in determining the location of a brain injury. Damage to any part of the reflex arc will cause a loss of that reflex. This injury may be to the spinal cord at the level of the reflex arc, to its afferent or efferent nerve, or to the muscle itself. An upper neurone lesion indicates an injury to the brain stem. This would cause reflexes that have centers below the level of the lesion to be hyperactive due to loss of control from the higher centers. An upper motor neurone lesion can be substantiated by a positive Babinski on the affected side.

Vital Signs

While the vital signs cannot pinpoint the exact area of brain injury, they are general indicators of such injury. When a head injury occurs blood pressure changes, with an increase in the systolic pressure coupled with a decrease in the diastolic pressure. The difference in these two readings is called the pulse pressure, and when the pulse pressure becomes higher than the pulse rate, there is danger of respiratory complications.[22] The first sign of such complications is a retardation of respiration, followed by irregular breathing, and finally by Cheyne-Stokes respirations, which consist of periods of rapid respirations that slow down and eventually cease entirely, only to repeat the cycle. The presence of Cheyne-Stokes respirations is the sign that respiratory failure is imminent and immediate emergency treatment is imperative.

Intracranial pressure should be suspected when any one or all of the following findings are present: (1) initially elevated blood pressure followed by a gradual drop in pressure; (2) a slowed, bounding pulse rate that gradually quickens; and (3) a rise in temperature followed by pulmonary edema. Severe headaches, dizziness, and/or vomiting may be a sign of increased intracranial pressure. Vomiting may produce serious consequences since it increases venous pressure, which in turn causes an increase in intracranial pressure. In addition, the unconscious athlete may aspirate the vomitus, resulting in pulmonary problems. Increased intracranial pressure may also cause seizures or twitching.[12] These symptoms occur early, shortly after a brain contusion or a depressed skull fracture. Seizures occurring later are more likely to be the result of hematomas and may develop a few hours to several days after injury, although in actuality they occur in less than 10 percent of the head-injury patients.

Neck rigidity is sometimes found in athletes receiving a head injury and may be caused by either an injury to the neck or by a hemorrhage in the subarachnoid space. Drainage of blood or clear fluid from the ears or nose is indicative of a basilar skull fracture or a fracture to the paranasal sinuses. Because these fractures tear the membranes covering the brain, the brain is thus exposed to infection. These leaking orifices should not be packed but should be allowed to drain freely and be cared for by a neurosurgeon.

MANAGEMENT OF A HEAD INJURY

The decision as to whether to allow an athlete to continue to play after he has received a head injury is a difficult one to make, since intracranial bleeding can occur gradually and observation during the first twelve hours post-injury can be critical. The decision ultimately depends upon an assessment of the severity of the injury, which is directly related to the duration and level of consciousness and to the existence and extent of retrograde and post-traumatic amnesia. Any player who has received a head injury, no matter how slight, should be removed from the game, at least temporarily, for further observation. If a player loses consciousness for just a few seconds or is momentarily dazed but experiences no memory loss, responds to questions about his assignments of play, and shows no residual ill effects, he can be returned to the game by the team physician.[13] This athlete must, however, be carefully observed on the field, with his performance and agility compared to his pre- and post-injury. Any variation in these comparisons indicates that the player should be removed from the game for further observation. Any player who has been unconscious for longer than a minute, and who has periods of amnesia, must be closely examined periodically for localizing signs, muscle strength and coordination, and for evidence of long-lasting amnesia. These observations and measurements are best taken while the athlete is sitting on the bench rather than being sent to the training room, where close observation is difficult. When any symptoms have completely subsided, the athlete is asked to run along the sidelines and is quizzed on his assignments in various plays. All of these tests are repeated in order to determine if there has been an improvement in his condition. The physician will then decide either to return the athlete to the game or to keep him under close observation. It is important to bear in mind that the athletes are young and healthy and have excellent powers of recuperation. More often than not, the injuries sustained on the field have no long-lasting effects.

It is crucial that the physician be able to evaluate each player individually, understanding that one athlete's intense desire to return to the game may cause him to minimize his symptoms, while another may be overly concerned about his injury and tend to maximize his symptoms. In one game several years ago, two athletes received head impacts and were removed from the game. One player said that there was nothing wrong with him and requested that he be returned to the game, while the other was very concerned about his injury, repeatedly asking that his pulse and pupils be checked. Examination of the first player revealed that he was suffering from a headache that was aggravated by motion, although he denied any problem, and he was removed from the game. The other player was physically able to return to the game, but his mental agitation over his perceived injury made his return impossible.

An athlete who has been unconscious for a period of two to five minutes has received a serious concussion and should not, under any circumstances, be allowed to return to the game. Any loss of consciousness beyond five minutes definitely requires hospitalization and careful observation.[5] It is important that this player must not be given pain killers to relieve his symptoms, since narcotics, tranquilizers, or barbiturates will depress his respiration and may mask the symptoms of head injury.

SUMMARY

The proper identification and management of head injuries resulting on the playing field is the most important responsibility of the medical team. Above all, the medical team should not cause further injury to an unconscious player by moving him prior to an on-field total body evaluation, with any life-threatening symptoms treated on the spot. Following this, the medical team must begin a detailed and systematic recording of the player's level of consciousness, eye signs, and muscle action. During the time the medical team is making these notations, the athlete should regain consciousness, begin to carefully move his head, sit up, and finally be able to walk off the field. If such a recovery does not occur and the medical team has completed its evaluation, a litter will be required to transport the player to the sidelines.

Regardless of the severity of an injury, the detailed post-injury report compiled by the medical team will prove invaluable, particularly in the case of an athlete who must be rushed to the hospital. In such a situation, the record and evaluations made by the medical team will save the hospital physician precious time and aid him in his diagnosis and treatment of the injured athlete.

REFERENCES

1. Bell, J. A.: Eye trauma in sports: a preventable epidemic. *JAMA, 246*:156, 1981.
2. Clare, F. B., and Bell, H. S.: Epidural or extradural hematomas. *JAMA, 177*:887, 1961.
3. Corales, R. L., Maull, K. I., and Becker, D. P.: Phencyclidine abuse mimicking head injury. *JAMA, 243*:2323, 1980.
4. Corsellis, J. A. N.: Quoted in *Lancet,* Brain Damage in sports, *Feb. 21*:401, 1976.
5. Eisenbeiss, J. A.: Emergency diagnostic considerations. Classification of head injuries. *Seminar on Management of Head Injuries Conference Proceedings.* Phoenix, AZ: The Barrow Neurologic Institute, St. Joseph's Hospital, Nov. 24–25, 1967, p. 129.
6. Eliasoph, I.: Eyes get hurt too. *Bul Amer Coll Surg,* Oct. 11, 1981.
7. Goff, C. W., and Aldes, J. H.: The acute traumatic cervical syndrome. *Medical Science, April*:40, 1964.
8. Gronwall, D., and Wrightson, P.: Cumulative effect of concussion. *Lancet, No. 2*:995, 1975.
9. Hussey, H.: Punch drunk. *JAMA, 236*:485, 1976.
10. McCown, I. A.: Boxing safety and injuries. *The Physician and Sports Medicine, 7*:75, 1979.
11. McLaurin, R. L.: Answers to questions on head injuries. *Hospital Medicine, Jan.*:54, 1969.
12. Roberts, A. H.: Quoted in *Lancet,* Brain damage in sports, *Feb. 21*:401, 1976.
13. Ryan, A. J.: On-field diagnosis of head injuries. *The Physician and Sports Medicine, 4*:82, 1976.
14. Salibi, B. S.: Level of consciousness in acute head injuries. *CMD,* Jan., 1964 (Condensed from *Wisc Med J, 62*:375, 1963).
15. Sayers, M. P.: Acute football injuries of the brain and spinal cord. *Ohio State Med J, Aug*:895, 1961.
16. Schmidek, H. H.: Compications may arise in seconds — or months. *The Physician and Sports Medicine, 4*:68, 1976.
17. Schneider, R. C.: *Head and Neck Injuries in Football: Mechanism, Treatment, and Presentation.* Baltimore, Williams & Wilkins, 1973, p 17.
18. Sercl, M., and Jaros, O.: Mechanisms of cerebral concussion in boxing and their consequences. *World Neurol, 25*:183, 1962.
19. Standard Nomenclature of Athletic Injuries. Subcommittee on Classification of Sports Injuries, Committee of Medical Aspects of Sports. AMA, 1966, p. 20.
20. Stuteville, O. H.: Treatment of ear injuries. *The Official National Collegiate Athletic Association. Wrestling Guide.* New York, Barnes, 1948, p. 5.
21. Weinstoek, F. J.: Contact lenses. *JAMA, 246*:161, 1981.
22. Wilkins, H.: Craniocerebral injuries in athletes. In O'Donoghue, D. H.: *Treatment of Injuries to Athletes,* 2nd Ed., Philadelphia, Saunders, 1970, p. 103.

Chapter 10

IDENTIFICATION AND
MANAGEMENT OF NECK INJURIES

Less than half of the major cervical spine injuries involving fractures and dislocations result in spinal cord damage, but in that group of injuries where cord injury occurs, 4 percent to 7 percent are sports related.[7,14,16] Clark reported the incidence of permanent spinal cord injuries for the years 1973 through 1975 in 17,000 high school, junior college, and college athletes to be 64, 5, and 17, respectively.[5] Schneider[14] reported 78 cord injuries nationally for the years 1959 to 1963, and Torg[15] reported 12 cases in two states for the year 1975. Because of the potential for permanent damage, it is essential that any spinal injury be properly identified and managed to minimize its severity.[6]

The neck is the link between the head and body that houses the delicate tissue of the spinal cord, peripheral nerves, large blood vessels, and the trachea. The neck is composed of seven cervical vertebrae connected to one another by ligaments and supported by muscles and tendons, which permit a wide range of motion while also protecting these vital structures from injury. There are eight cervical nerve roots, the first root appearing in the interval between the skull and the first vertebra, and the eighth cervical root appearing between the seventh cervical and the first thoracic vertebrae. The number of the root corresponds to the space above the vertebra of the same number (i.e. the fifth nerve root leaves the spine in the space between C_4 and C_5). Peripheral nerves emanate from these cervical roots to form the cervical and brachial plexuses.

The cervical plexus is composed of the first four cervical nerve roots. It supplies innervation to the upper neck and head and is almost entirely sensory in function. The brachial plexus is a network of nerves formed from the lower four nerve roots of the cervical cord and the first thoracic nerve root. These five nerve roots join to form trunks, divide again to form cords, and divide once more to form identifiable peripheral nerves (Fig. 10-1).

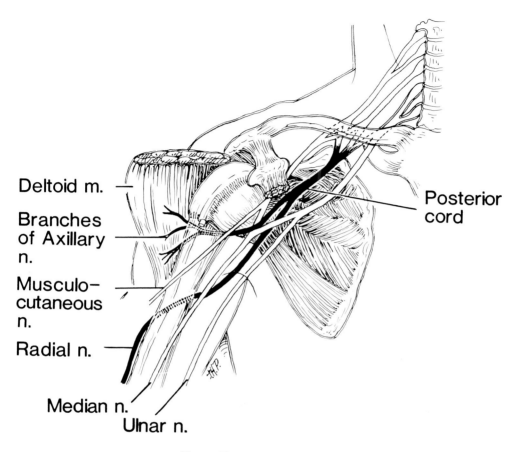

Deltoid m.

Branches
of Axillary
n.

Musculo-
cutaneous
n.

Radial n.

Median n.

Ulnar n.

Posterior
cord

Figure 10-1. Brachial plexus.

NECK INJURIES

Pharyngeal Injuries

Direct injury to the neck is uncommon because of its protected position and occurs only when a missile or other object strikes the neck. If this does occur, an injury to the larynx may result.[2] Consider the case of a player whose pharynx is injured when a baseball strikes his neck. Increasing airway obstruction occurs with stridor and difficulty breathing. Difficulty in talking follows with eventual aphonia. The player then coughs and may cough up or vomit swallowed blood. Neck pain increases and finally the athlete has difficulty swallowing. Bleeding may occur into the deep structures of the neck or escape of air from the trachea may cause respiratory difficulty requiring hospitalization. In severe cases a tracheostomy may have to be performed as an emergency measure. Any patient who requires a tracheostomy following neck trauma is presumed to have laryngeal trauma and must be referred to an otolaryngologist.

In the absence of pharyngeal injury, injury to the neck muscles or blood vessels may result in brisk bleeding and lead to hematoma formation. Because the muscles of the neck are encased in deep fascia, the bleeding will be confined to a closed compartment and may cause tracheal compression and subsequent respiratory distress. Releasing the pressure by opening the fascia can result in uncontrolled bleeding and must only be performed in the hospital.

It is important to note that in any attempt to control neck bleeding, pressure on the trachea must be avoided. Furthermore, pressure that restricts venous return will tend to increase rather than decrease bleeding. The method of treatment for such injuries is direct pressure over the injury site.

Potentially Serious Injuries

Neck injuries are more commonly the indirect result of a blow to the head or torso of an athlete and are most likely to occur at the point of maximum mobility adjacent to a relatively immobile section of the cervical spine.[6] The direction of the blow with regard to the long axis of the cervical spine determines the type of injury.

The athlete who spears aligns his cervical spine in the direction of the blow. This causes the entire counterforce to be exerted by the bony spine. Great compressive force is borne by the soft cancellous bone of the vertebral bodies. Because muscles and ligaments act merely to splint the spine, they are infrequently injured. Fractures more commonly occur and may range from a simple chip off the corner of the anterior border of the body of a vertebra, anterior wedging of the entire anterior border, or a complete destruction of a vertebral body with attendant spinal cord damage.

A blow striking the head at an angle to the long axis of the cervical spine will put the head into sudden motion independent of the body and will strain the neck as its range of motion is exceeded. This type of injury more likely involves ligaments and the intervertebral joints. Because the force of the blow has some compressive action, some bony injury may occur. Depending upon the magnitude of the force, this bony injury may be quite severe and include avulsion of the components of the neural arch. A severe flexion injury was received by an eighteen-year-old freshman football player at Northwestern University when he lowered his head in tackling. His opponent's knee struck the back of his helmet, forcing his neck into extreme flexion. Following the blow, he lay on the ground complaining of feeling very warm and unable to move the fingers of his right hand or extend his right elbow. On examination he was found to have good deltoid and biceps function, but he had no movement below the level of C_6. In addition, hyperactive deep tendon reflexes were noted in the lower extremities. He was transported to the hospital where AP and lateral x-rays of his cervical spine were taken, revealing an anterior dislocation of C_4 on C_5 (Fig. 10-2). No fractures were demonstrated. He was placed in immediate skeletal traction using Crutchfield tongs. On the following day right-arm function returned, with some associated movement of the right triceps muscle. It was determined that surgery was necessary, during which it was revealed that bilateral fractures of the lamina of C_5 had occurred, with complete separation of the spinous process from its body. The dislocation had been spontaneously reduced, but the posterior longitudinal ligament had ruptured, allowing the disc to project into the canal. The surgeon removed the disc and fused the area. An anterior fusion of the vertebral bodies was subsequently required. After a long hospitalization, the athlete was discharged with only some residual weakness of the triceps muscle of the right arm.

If the force to the head is disruptive, such as occurs when a player grasps the face mask of his opponent and attempts to pull his head away from his body, bony damage is unlikely but ligamentous strain may be so severe that a complete disruption of the intervertebral joint may occur. This can result in a subluxation of the joint, which may reduce spontaneously and leave no x-ray evidence of the serious nature of this injury.

Whiplash Injuries

The neck may be injured when the body is unexpectedly driven into motion while the inert head stays behind as occurs with a whiplash injury. This type of flexion action, when coupled with rotary motion, can cause a subluxation of the joint on one side of the neck as the inferior articular facet slides up and over the superior facet of the vertebra below. Subluxation can occur with very little associated ligament strain, with the subluxation locked in an unreduced position. An example of this involved an injury received by a nineteen-year-old freshman split end who had been tackled while receiving a forward pass. On examination, tenderness of the right sternocleidomastoid muscle was noted. Although there were no positive neurologic findings, the athlete was unable to extend his neck. We suspected a potentially serious neck injury, and the player was sent for x-rays, where a subluxation of C_3 on C_4 on the right side only was demonstrated (Fig. 10-3). Marked spasm and tenderness persisted and so the athlete was taken to surgery. The subluxation of the faceted joint was reduced and stabilized with no sequelae.

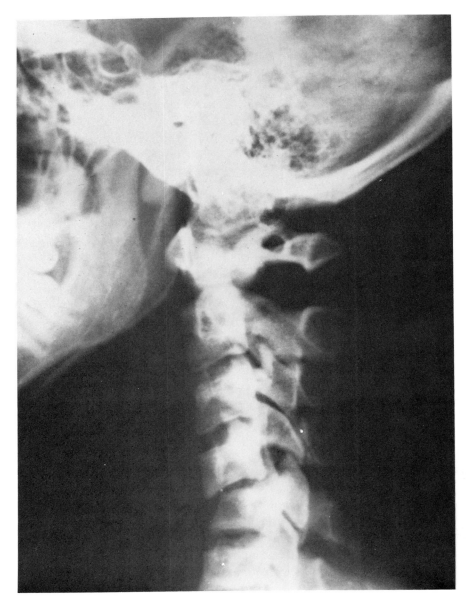

Figure 10-2. Anterior dislocation C_4 on C_5.

Brachial Plexus Injuries

Injuries involving the brachial plexus are very common in football.[3,4,12] During the 1980 season and the 1981 spring practice of the Northwestern

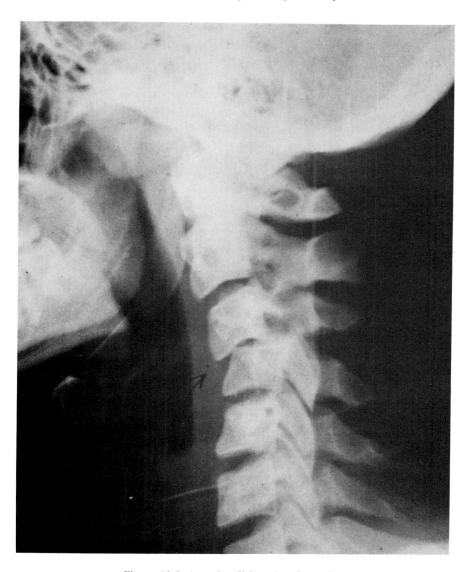

Figure 10-3. Anterior dislocation C_3 on C_4.

University football team, 37 varsity players received a total of 115 brachial plexus injuries. One player received eight such injuries; eleven players suffered three injuries each. Fifteen of the injured athletes playing on the defensive secondary received 54 brachial plexus injuries; 11 defensive linemen were injured 36 times. Although the majority of these injuries were minor, they did necessitate removing the athlete from at least one series of play. Furthermore, recurrences were common following the initial injury; in only six players was the injury a one-time occurrence, and each recurrent injury was generally more severe than the original. Each injury resulted in the loss of playing time, although all did heal with no residual effects.

Forced lateral flexion of the cervical spine may cause injury to the brachial plexus in three ways: (1) stretching, (2) pinching, and (3) direct pressure to any part of the plexus. Stretching injuries are caused when the neck is forced to the side, thereby increasing the span traversed by the upper trunk of the plexus. This stretching will be increased if the shoulder is also depressed by the impact, with the result that the C_5 and C_6 nerve roots, the upper trunk, and the peripheral nerves emanating from these roots will be subjected to the greatest stretch of the entire brachial plexus (Fig. 10-4).[4,17]

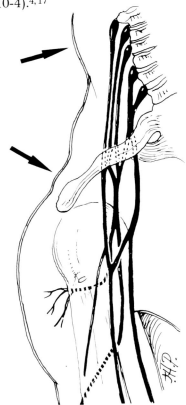

Figure 10-4. Stretched brachial plexus, especially the axillary nerve.

Pinching injuries of the brachial plexus are also the result of lateral flexion of the head, which causes the chin to rotate toward the side of flexion. When this occurs the intervertebral foramen, which is normally twice the size of the nerve root, the blood vessels, and the dural sleeve that pass through the foramen, is narrowed on the side opposite the blow, pinching the nerve root, particularly at the point of maximum flexion: the C_5–C_6 interspace (Fig. 10-5). Repeated trauma is likely to cause arthritic changes, further reducing the size of the foramen and doing more damage to the sixth nerve root.

Pressure injuries to the brachial plexus resulting from lateral flexion may be caused by improperly fitted shoulder pads whose supporting straps are too close to the root of the neck. This pressure may also exaggerate the stretching of the plexus when the head is forced to the side and the shoulder is depressed. A ruptured disc resulting from the forced lateral flexion of the cervical spine can also cause pressure on a cervical nerve root of the brachial plexus, and although this is a less common cause of a pressure injury, it does occur. Even a small rupture of the disc can cause severe pressure due to the relative immobility of the cervical nerve root within the confined space of the intervertebral foramen.

Another possible cause of brachial plexus injury occurs in the well-muscled athlete at the point where the trunks of the brachial plexus leave the neck.[17] This occurs immediately above the medial third of the clavicle in the cleft formed between the two hypertrophied and actively contracting scalene anterior and medius muscles and their insertion on the first rib (Fig. 10-6). Entrapment of the nerves by these muscles is likely and is similar to the situation that exists when the paravertebral muscles of the neck compromise the greater occipital nerve, causing pain in the occiput and vertex of the skull.

Two significant brachial plexus injuries occurred during our thirty years experience with the Northwestern University football team. The first involved a twenty-year-old defensive tackle with a well-developed neck who had had three previous episodes of brachial plexus injury, with each successive injury being more severe than the previous one. A head-on collision with the helmet of another player caused his head to be deflected down and to the left. Immediately following impact, his left arm was limp and numb and he experienced severe left neck pain. The pain instantaneously moved down beneath his left scapula, to the small of his back, down the posterior aspect of his left arm, across the elbow, and down the anterior surface of his forearm to his three middle fingers. After about fifty minutes he was able to move his left arm, although marked muscle weakness was noted. Physical examination revealed decreased biceps and triceps reflexes and strength on the left side and a weakened hand grasp. The Babinski test on the left side was positive, and sensation to pinprick was diminished on the posterior aspect of his left arm, forearm, midpalm, and middle three fingers. Examination the following day revealed that the strength of all muscles innervated by the C_6 and T_1 roots was reduced and reflexes on the left side were weak. Knee jerks were brisk, with the left being slightly greater than the right, and a questionable Babinski on the left side with an unsustained clonus at the

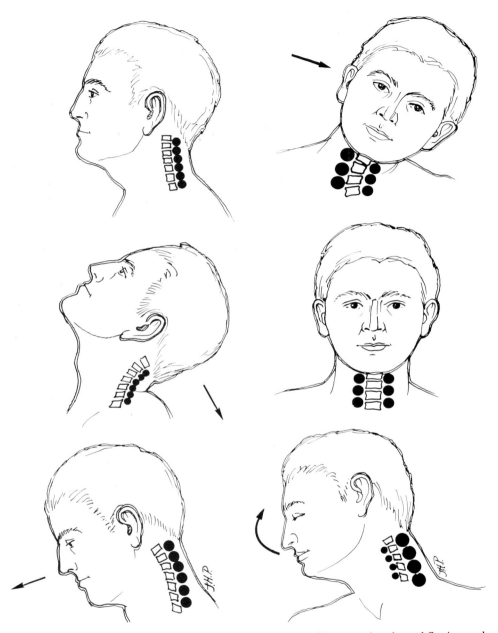

Figure 10-5. The size of the intervertebral foramina is reduced in extension, lateral flexion and rotation of the neck.

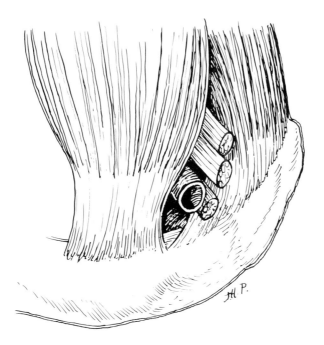

Figure 10-6. Hypertrophied scalene anterior and medius muscle inserting on the first rib could be an explanation for a brachial plexus pinch as these nerves escape in the cleft between these muscles.

ankle was observed. A myelogram defined the injury as limited to the brachial plexus, with a probable traction injury of the cervical roots, rather than a herniated disc and transient cord compression. This injury completely healed over a twelve-month period, but the athlete was not permitted to return to the team.

The second serious brachial plexus injury involved a defensive guard who was injured tackling a ball carrier. He immediately experienced sharp pain over the left chest and shoulder, which radiated down his left arm to the hand and fingertips. He also noted transient numbness and weakness of the right arm and hand. The pain was aggravated by any movement of his head when his chin pointed to the left side. He continued to play out the rest of the season, during which time the symptoms subsided, leaving only some residual weakness of his left hand. During the spring practice the next year, however, following a tackle that forced his neck into acute right lateral flexion, he experienced sharp pain over his right shoulder that traveled down his arm to the tips of his fingers. The pain was so severe that he was unable to move his right arm. Subsequently, the pain decreased, but it recurred when he turned his head toward the affected side. Weakness of his right hand and arm persisted, and he could not extend his elbow against the resistance provided by the examiner's finger. In addition, the grip of the right hand was weak, and he experienced numbness of the right index finger and weakness of the right hand for two to three weeks. He experienced no associated headaches or dizziness, and his left upper extremity was asymptomatic. Forward flexion of the neck was normal, but restricted motion on flexion and extension of the neck to the right was noted. Because of the continued weakness and pain along the distribution of the median nerve, a diagnosis of a herniated disc was made. In addition, post-traumatic osteoarthritic lipping of C_5 and C_6 vertebrae bilaterally caused by previous injuries was noted. A bilateral hemilaminectomy of C_5 and C_6 was performed, and the surgery demonstrated a marked bilateral overlapping of the lamina of C_5 over C_6, particularly on the right side. The sixth right cervical nerve root appeared flattened, but there was no disc injury. The root was decompressed, and one week later there was no pain associated with head rotation, although the numbness in the fingers persisted. The injury eventually became asymptomatic.

EXAMINATION FOR NECK INJURY

Neck injuries occur in approximately 5 percent to 10 percent of all unconscious players, and any neck injury must be considered a part of the head injury complex. It is important to note that while at least 50 percent of all neck fractures and dislocations involve no cord injury, a paralyzing spinal cord injury can be caused by hasty movement of the injured athlete. It is imperative that the athlete be examined in the position in which he is found. As we have mentioned previously, this initial on-field examination does not require helmet removal, since the helmet helps to support the head and its removal could cause further damage to the already injured neck.

Examination of the neck consists of carefully observing the position of the neck for signs of dislocation. Any swelling should be noted, as well as the degree of patient discomfort. The athlete should be questioned about previous neck injuries and asked about the mechanism of this injury. He should then be questioned about the location of his pain. Radiation of pain into the interscapular area or down into the arm and/or fingers needs to be recorded. The ability of the athlete to move all four extremities must be determined at this time. Evidence of a hematoma or an ecchymosis over the bony prominences of the spine or immediately lateral to the spine in the extensor muscles should be noted, as well as any disparity in the distances between the spinous processes. Because considerable apprehension usually accompanies this type of injury, it is important to reassure the athlete that he will not be subjected to any unnecessary pain during the examination and that the examination and questions are essential in order to avoid serious injury.

Increased muscle tone is evidence of spasm. Spasm is accompanied by pain and tenderness, generally in the region of the posterior cervical muscles, and neck motion will aggravate the pain.[10] If the athlete persists in holding his head to one side, the examiner should immediately recognize that the neck muscles are in spasm and be on the alert for the cause of this spasm. Dizziness, blurred vision, unsteady gait, nausea, and tinnitus are often associated with spasm of the posterior cervical musculature and may be the result of circulatory impairment in the last two inches of the vertebral artery as it passes from the transverse process of C_2 up into the brain through the foramen magnum. Numbness or tingling in the back of the head that radiates to the top and sides of the head is probably the result of a stretching or impingement of the greater occipital nerve, which is also caused by muscle spasm.

The ability of the athlete to move his neck should be determined by passive motion. This is accomplished by the physician gently flexing, extending, and rotating the neck while the athlete is questioned about any pain or change in sensation in his extremities. The entire procedure must be performed very carefully and without force. Evidence of pain or change in sensation is a warning signal to stop any further motion. Neck motion should be tested in all directions. When the athlete feels secure, and if movement has not caused any radiation of pain, the athlete should then be asked to gently flex his own neck, touching his chin to his chest. When active motion is possible, the athlete is asked to try to sit up. If he can do this, he is allowed to try to stand. Provided he has no problem standing, he can walk off the field. If during the preliminary tests there is any evidence of a more serious injury such as the suspicion of a neurologic deficit, marked spasm of the neck muscles, limitation of neck motion, pain caused by the slightest motion, or referral of pain or numbness into the extremities, the player must be treated with extreme care and possibly removed from the field by litter. The player must be slowly and gently eased on to the litter, with his head supported and immobilized during the entire procedure.

The most common cause of immediate paralysis following trauma is spinal cord shock.[13] This is a temporary concussion of the cord and does not result in permanent paralysis. Spinal cord shock, nevertheless, must be treated as though it were an actual compression of the cord. The crucial point to remember here is that an athlete who has had any degree of limited neck motion must be considered to have a more serious injury and treated as such until further diagnostic studies demonstrate otherwise. As we have previously mentioned, in this situation no attempts should be made to change the position of the head and neck. If there should be any need for slight motion of the neck, the position of slight extension is the position of choice. This relies on the fact that the anterior longitudinal ligament, which is rarely injured, splints the anterior part of the spine and properly aligns the vertebrae when the head and neck are slightly extended (Fig. 10-7).

One question that is frequently asked is whether traction should be applied to the head while the injured athlete is being transported on the litter. The answer to this question is usually no. First of all, the exact amount of traction necessary would be hard to maintain in a well-muscled athlete. Secondly, it would be very difficult to maintain this traction during transport. Finally, traction is essentially unnecessary, since the muscle spasm that exists after injury will tend to splint the neck, thereby protecting the cord. During transport, the head and neck should be supported with rolled towels or sandbags and the helmet can be secured to the litter with adhesive tape (Fig. 10-8). Remember that the helmet is to be left on until the player arrives at the hospital. At that time it must be removed in a definitely prescribed manner in order to avoid doing further injury to the cervical spine.[8]

IDENTIFICATION OF NECK INJURIES

As we mentioned earlier, brachial plexus injuries are quite common in football, and early differentiation of such an injury from a cervical spine injury is necessary. The athlete who is standing or walking on the field in obvious pain, with his arm hanging limply at his side, is clearly suffering from a brachial plexus injury. The radiation of sharp, burning pain in the upper extremity confirms the diagnosis of nerve, rather than muscle injury. When questioned, the athlete will be able to describe the extent of pain radiation, which may be felt in the base of the neck, extending into the trapezius and deltoid muscles, and radiate into the arm, forearm, and hand. This sharp pain radiation, which is referred to as the physiologic portion of the injury, will subside within a few minutes, becoming a dull ache in the region of the neck and shoulder.

The multiple mechanism involved in brachial plexus trauma, combined with the complex distribution of nerve roots to the various components of the plexus, make the physical diagnosis of the injury to a specific nerve root extremely difficult. The following is a description of the contributions of each of the five roots of the brachial plexus.

C_5 — Deltoid, biceps, supraspinatus and infraspinatus muscles. Other muscles also supplied include rhomboid, brachialis, and the clavicular head of the pectoralis major muscle.

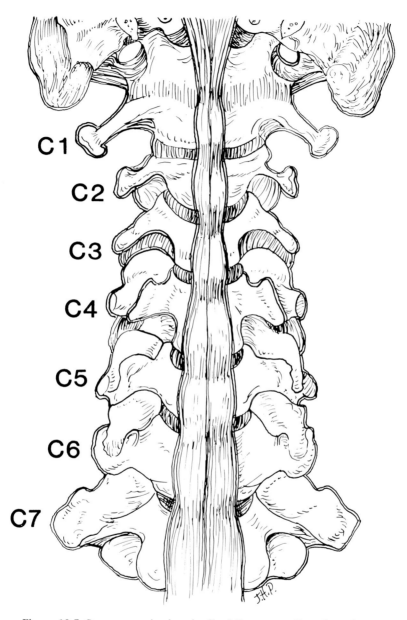

C1

C2

C3

C4

C5

C6

C7

Figure 10-7. Strong anterior longitudinal ligament splints the spine.

C_6— Triceps. Another muscle supplied is the sternal head of the pectoralis major muscle.

C_7— Extensors of the wrist and fingers.

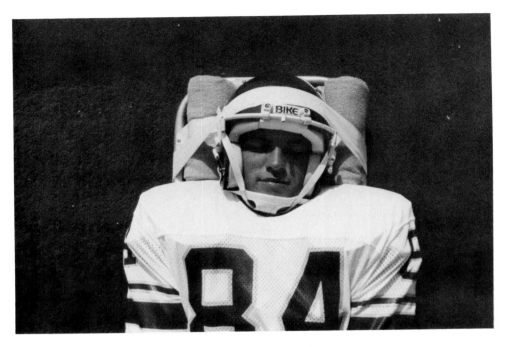

Figure 10-8. Helmet taped to litter during transport.

C_8 — Flexors of the wrist and fingers.
T_1 — Intrinsic muscles of the hand, for finer movements, and the cervical sympathetics.

The sensory distribution of the nerves to the head and neck is given in Figure 10-9.

Very little neck muscle spasm is associated with injuries to the brachial plexus. This fact is helpful in diagnosing specific brachial plexus injuries because the neck can be moved into lateral flexion until pain occurs, whereupon the point of trauma can then be localized. In attempting to diagnose these specific nerve root injuries, it is important to keep in mind that the C_5 and C_6 nerve roots are most commonly injured in football, whereas the lower portion of the plexus (C_7, C_8, and T_1) is rarely affected. When such an injury does occur, it is usually minor in nature, with spontaneous recovery. An injury to the axillary nerve of the C_5 root is demonstrated by a weakness of the deltoid muscle, coupled with diminished sensation to the skin overlying the lower portion of this muscle. Injury to the musculocutaneous nerves— another component of the C_5 root—will produce weakness of the biceps muscle, diminished biceps reflex, weakness of the elbow flexion, and weakness of forearm pronation. When the radial nerve, which is a component in

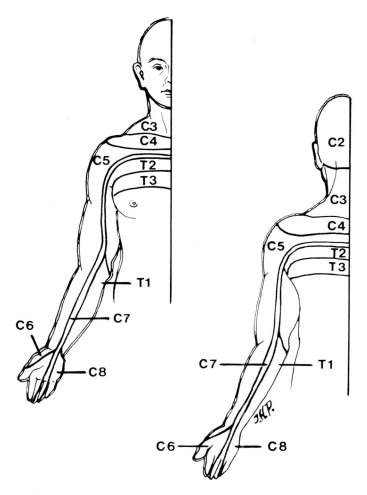

Figure 10-9. Sensory distribution of nerves to head and neck.

the C_6 root, is injured, there will be evidence of weakness of the triceps muscle in elbow extension, diminished triceps reflex, and weakness of forearm supination (Fig. 10-10).

A blow to the forehead may result in a bilateral brachial plexus nerve root pinch caused by subsequent compressing of the neck, which forces it into hyperextension. Symptoms of this condition are a feeling of deadness in both upper extremities in conjunction with a burning pain radiating down both arms, with *no involvement of lower extremities*. The arm paralysis lasts only about a minute, but the pain continues, although it may be somewhat diminished. It should be noted that the radiation of pain does not necessarily extend to the same level in both arms. The side of the greater pain

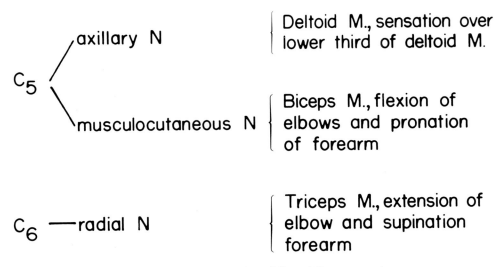

Figure 10-10. Shows function of C₅ and C₆ nerve roots.

radiation usually has received a more severe injury, and the symptoms of that side will persist longer.

MANAGEMENT OF A NECK INJURY

Both the athlete who is able to walk off the field and the player who is removed by litter must undergo further examination on the sidelines or in the training room unless taken directly to the hospital. Examination on the sidelines should re-evaluate the on-field findings, noting any changes that may have occurred with regard to pain, stiffness, and headache. Progression in any symptoms must be followed in the training room, where sensory and motor changes elicited by pinprick and deep reflex function should be tested. It is imperative that an athlete be withdrawn from play until all signs of restricted neck motion have subsided. Spasm of the cervical musculature may merely be the result of muscle strain or sprain, but it can also indicate a more serious injury such as a subluxation of the articular facets resulting from minor ligament strain or derangement of a posterior intervertebral joint caused by severe ligamentous injury. Such an injury may be demonstrated radiographically by cervical spine straightening. A small chip fracture of the anterior surface of the body of the vertebra may be the only indication of severe ligamentous injury and subluxation of intervertebral joints that have spontaneously reduced.

Immobilizing the neck with a collar can help to alleviate the strain on a ligament and minimize muscle spasm by supporting the weight of the head, but the collar should be worn during the acute phase of injury only. Once this phase has passed, exercise should be initiated in order to improve circulation of the injured muscles and to prevent edema.

Neck traction is not indicated in the acute phase following a whiplash injury, nor should it be used when marked spasm and tenderness persist, since these are signs of ligamentous injury.[10] If there is an indication of nerve involvement upon physical examination, however, gentle traction may be helpful once any spasm has subsided.

The treatment of brachial plexus injuries depends upon their severity. Acute conditions may be alleviated by holding the extremity in a sling or by keeping the neck immobilized in a collar. Ice packs should be applied to the injury for fifteen to twenty minutes, three or four times a day for the first forty-eight hours, and periodic examination should be performed to determine the persistence of tenderness and restricted motion. After the first forty-eight hours, neck exercises should be initiated, beginning with passive exercises, moving on to active motion, and finally having the athlete flex and extend his neck against resistance. When the athlete is ready to return to the team, it is important to take precautions against re-injury. These precautions include continued exercises for muscular strength in the neck and checking the shoulder pads to make certain they do not press on the plexus. Occasionally, recurrent injury may be avoided by merely moving a lineman to the other side of the scrimmage line so as to alter the direction of any future blows.

SUMMARY

We cannot overemphasize the importance of proper identification and management by the medical team of neck injuries occurring on the football field. Although most football-related neck injuries are not of a catastrophic variety, an iatrogenic paralyzing spinal cord injury can result from the hasty movement of an injured athlete. As we discussed in the previous chapter as well as in this one, the medical team must begin evaluating an injury while the player is still on the field, maintaining careful records of all findings. Once the player has been removed to the sidelines, the evaluation procedure continues. Finally, it is the responsibility of the medical team to make absolutely certain that no athlete returns to the game until he has totally recovered from the serious effects of his neck injury.

REFERENCES

1. Allen, A. R.: Surgery of experimental lesion of the spinal cord equivalent to crush injury of fracture dislocation of the spinal column. *JAMA, 57*:878, 1911.
2. Ballenger, J. J.: *Diseases of the Nose, Throat and Ear,* 12th Ed., Philadelphia, Lea, 1977.
3. Chrisman, O. D., Snook, G. A., Stanitis, J. M., and Keedy, V. A.: Lateral flexion neck injuries in athletic competition. *JAMA, 192*:613, 1965.
4. Clancy, W. G., Brand, R. L., and Bergfeld, J. A.: Upper trunk brachial plexus injury in contact sports. *J Sports Med, 5*:209, 1977.
5. Clark, K. S.: A survey of sports related spinal cord injuries in schools and colleges. *J Safety Res, 9*:140, 1977.
6. Clark, K.: Injuries to the cervical spine and spinal cord. In Youmans, J. R. (Ed.): *Neurological Surgery.* Philadelphia, Saunders, 1982.
7. Feldick, H. G., and Albright, J. P.: Football survey reveals missed neck injuries. *Physicians and Sports Med, 4*:77, 1976.
8. Long, S. E., Reid, S. E., Sweeney, H. J., and Johnson, W. W.: Removing football helmets safely. *Physicians and Sports Med, 8*:119, 1980.
9. Maroon, J. C.: Catastrophic neck injuries from football in Western Pennsylvania. *Physicians and Sports Med, 9*:783, 1981.
10. O'Donoghue, D. H.: *Treatment of Injuries to Athletes,* 2nd Ed. Philadelphia, Saunders, 1970.
11. Roaf, R.: Lateral flexion injuries of the cervical spine. *J Bone & Joint Surg, 45B*:36, 1963.
12. Robertson, W. C., Eichman, P. L., and Clancy, W. G.: Upper trunk brachial plexopathy in football players. *JAMA, 241*:1480, 1979.
13. Sayers, M. P.: Acute football injuries of the brain and spinal cord. *Ohio State Med J, Aug*:95, 1961.
14. Schneider, R. C.: *Head and Neck Injuries in Football.* Baltimore, Williams & Wilkins, 1973.
15. Torg, J. S., Quedenfeld, T. C., Burstein, A., Spealman, A., and Nichols, C., III: National Football Head and Neck Injury Registry: Report on cervical quadriplegia, 1971–1975. *Am J Sports Med, 7*:127, 1979.
16. Torg, J. S.: *Athletic Injuries to the Head, Neck and Face.* Philadelphia, Lea & Febiger, 1982.
17. Turek, S. L.: *Orthopedics Principles and Their Application,* 3rd Ed. Philadelphia, Lippincott, 1977.

Chapter 11

PREVENTION AND REHABILITATION
OF HEAD AND NECK INJURIES

One of the primary responsibilities of the medical team is to make certain that an athlete is totally prepared physically and mentally for the demands of the game. Should an injury occur, he must be protected against further injury, and a reconditioning program must be initiated as soon as possible following injury to return him to top form so that he may again participate in the sport. No shortcuts in the reconditioning process that could jeopardize a player's health or future well-being may be taken, although the motivation of a young, vigorous athlete generally makes rehabilitation a speedy process.

INJURY PREVENTION

There are many aspects to be considered when speaking of injury prevention, ranging from the selection of only those players who are physically suited for a particular sport, the enforcing of strict health standards, the requirement that all players be in top physical condition, the purchase of the best type of athletic equipment, and, finally, adherence to proper coaching techniques. Obviously, younger players should be grouped according to their size and maturity, bearing in mind that those players who are not yet fully developed must be excluded from vigorous contact sports. Regardless of an athlete's natural ability, he must also have the desire to play the sport. Once the individual decides he does wish to play football, for example, and assuming he seems physically suited to the sport, a complete physical examination is in order. This examination must include a history of previous injuries, with any previous neck injuries studied via x-rays of the cervical spine.[1] Any individual who has a history of multiple concussions should seriously consider changing from football to some other sport.

Physical Conditioning

A well-organized physical conditioning program can be the greatest determining factor in the prevention of injuries.[5,6] Conditioning of the athlete must be completed before he is allowed to participate in the game. Moreover, an athlete must maintain his physical conditioning program the year around so that he is able to report back at the beginning of the season ready for competition.[9] With respect to the neck, physical conditioning encompasses a wide variety of muscle development.

Flexibility Exercises

Range of motion exercises increase the flexibility of the neck, ensuring proper shoulder girdle and cervical spine flexibility to meet the demands of each specific sport. Lack of such flexibility can lead to injuries to nerves, ligaments, and muscle structures of the neck and surrounding areas.

There are a variety of range of motion exercises, including passive, active, active-assistive, and dynamic exercises.[2,10] Passive exercise of a joint is motion produced without any effort on the part of the athlete. It is accomplished by means of a machine or by another person moving the joint through its full range of motion. Active exercise involves the athlete himself moving a particular joint. Active-assistive exercise is movement initiated by the athlete, which is then aided by an external force, either a machine or another individual (Fig. 11-1). Dynamic exercise is active motion against resistance, such as the resistance of force or weights (Fig. 11-2).

As far as the conditioning process is concerned, the range of motion exercises are best performed in the active mode, where the athlete himself moves his head and neck through their complete range of motion without another person or machine forcing the neck beyond its normal range of motion (Fig. 11-3). In performing range of motion exercises, it is important that no one body area becomes more developed than another. The goal here is *total* body flexibility to aid in the prevention of possibly serious injuries.

Strengthening Exercises

The purpose of muscle-strengthening exercises is to provide the strength necessary to resist a blow, thereby preventing injury. It is important, however, that muscle strength is not developed at the expense of flexibility. The two must be balanced according to the needs of the particular sport.[4] A weight-training program should be followed the year round to build and maintain strength and flexibility. This program may follow several methods, one of which exclusively uses isometrics, which is resistance against an immovable object: for example, an athlete on his hands and knees attempting to extend his head against the resistance offered by an attendant who is holding the athlete's head in a fixed position (Fig. 11-4). The problem with isometrics, however, is that it builds strength in only one plane of motion and, therefore, does not provide total conditioning.

Another useful strength-training method involves isokinetics: a method

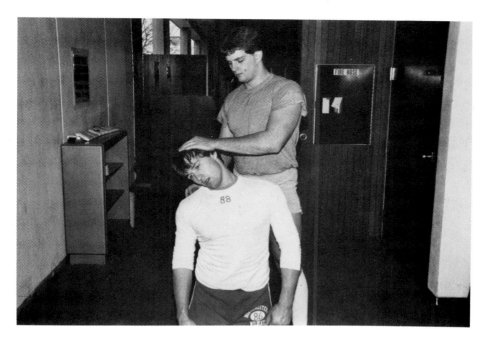

Figure 11-1. Active assist exercise. Motion by the athlete is assisted by another individual.

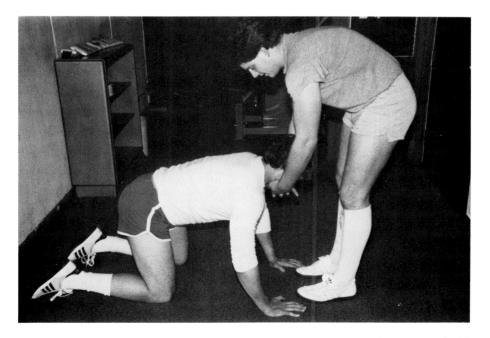

Figure 11-2. Dynamic exercise. Another individual offers resistance to active motion of athlete.

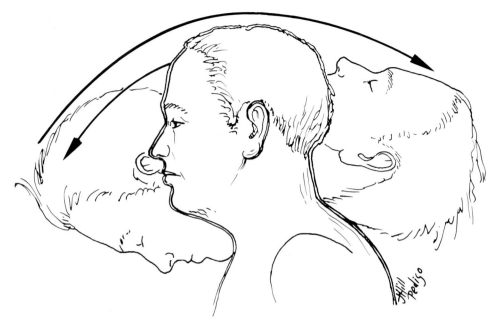

Figure 11-3. Unassisted range of motion exercise.

that utilizes varied resistance throughout the full range of motion. Isokinetics is accomplished with a machine that provides a controlled rate of shortening of a particular muscle while varying resistance. Unfortunately, there are very few cervical kinetic exercise programs, apparently due to the fact that the neck has a multiple, rather than a single, pivotal point of motion.

The method of weight training called isotonics utilizes the movement of weights to build strength. The Nautilus and Universal machines are examples of the isotonic principle. They have a four-way neck weight-training program that isolates the shoulder girdle and cervical spine to permit exercise in all four planes of neck motion: flexion, extension, and lateral movement. These machines have the ability to totally develop eccentric and concentric muscle activity. Eccentric muscle activity is negative work: the muscle actually lengthens during contraction when an external force or weight is applied. Concentric muscle activity is positive work: the muscle contracts, thereby moving the weight. Eccentric work builds strength at a slightly faster rate than does concentric work. A complete workout with the Nautilus or Universal machine should be done three times per week. We will describe such a program later in this chapter.

An athlete engaged in a year-round muscle-training program has to work not only on the cervical region but on the shoulder girdle itself. This is best

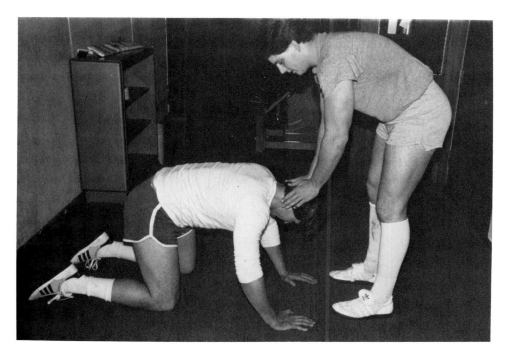

Figure 11-4. Isometric exercise. Extend neck against resistance.

accomplished by exercising the trapezius muscle doing shoulder shrugs, military presses, and two-iron curls. In shoulder shrugs, the trapezius muscle is exercised as the shoulders are raised toward the ears. This is performed while holding barbells of varying weights in downstretched arms, which provides resistance to shoulder movement (Fig. 11-5). When doing the military press, an athlete stands with his feet shoulder-width apart and raises the barbell from his chest over his head, completely extending his arms, then slowly lowers the barbell (Fig. 11-6). The two-arm curl is an exercise in which an athlete stands and grasps the barbell in the middle of the bar with his two hands together, raises the bar to his chin, then slowly lowers it to its original position (Fig. 11-7).

Another form of weight resistance for the cervical region involves a homemade device. A helmet is fitted with a bar on top of it to hold weights. The athlete puts on the helmet and lies down, going through the entire range of neck motion with a specific amount of weight fixed to the bar. Although this method will build muscle strength, it is not recommended for two important reasons: (1) neck muscles fatigue easily, and (2) because of muscle fatigue, the neck may be incapable of supporting the weight of the helmet and injury may result. In addition, since the weights are added at

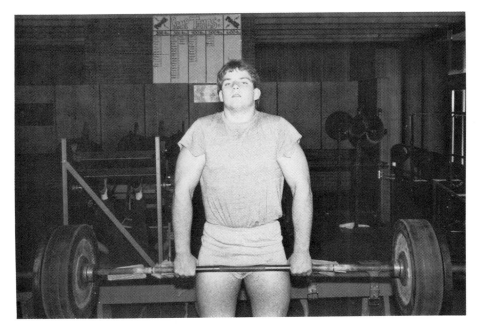

Figure 11-5. Exercise to strength trapezius muscles involve shoulder shrugs against resistance.

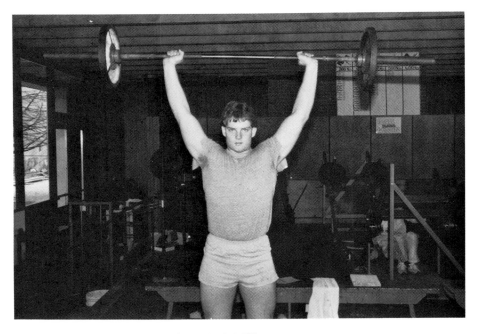

Figure 11-6. Military press.

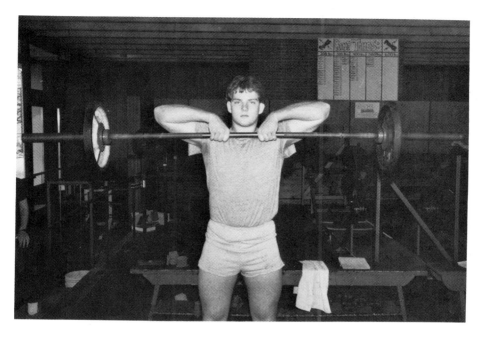

Figure 11-7. Two-arm curl.

increasing distances from the center of gravity, even greater strain is placed on these already fatigued muscles.

Isotonic Exercise Program

When beginning a program of progressive isotonic exercises, which is most effective when done using a Nautilus machine or similar apparatus, it is essential that the athlete perform fifteen minutes of warm-up exercise at the beginning and end of his workout. During this warm-up, the neck and shoulder girdle must be actively exercised throughout their full range of motion, making sure that the glenohumeral area and trapezius muscle are stretched. This stretching is necessary to prevent cervical strain and injury to the shoulder and brachial plexus. Warm-up exercises should employ light weights with five to ten repetitions of each exercise.[8]

When the warm-up is completed, the athlete moves on to the first Nautilus station. Being careful to maintain proper positioning and technique throughout, he will begin the first set with three sets of ten repetitions without weights (Fig. 11-8, 11-9, & 11-10). During the second and third sets, weights are added and the repetitions are decreased by one or two per set, depending upon the athlete and the amount of strength desired. During all of these exercises the body must be immobilized so that only the neck is being exercised. After using the Nautilus four-way neck machine, the athlete should perform shoulder shrugs to build up the trapezius and other neck muscles. Three sets of ten to twelve repetitions of shoulder shrugs should be done. At no time during this exercise program should neck bridging occur. Neck bridging involves the supine athlete arching his back, hyperextending his neck, and then raising his lower body, keeping his knees flexed, so that his entire weight is carried on his feet and head (Fig. 11-11). This places unnecessary stress on the intervertebral joints, which can result in damage to the articular facets. In any isotonic exercise program, neck exercises should always be performed first when the athlete is free from fatigue. He will then be able to concentrate on using proper technique and will not have to rest before completing the exercises. Development of upper-body musculature is an important part of this training program that is best accomplished with the Nautilus machine (Fig. 11-12, 11-13, 11-14, 11-15, & 11-16).

Endurance is an integral part of the isotonic bodybuilding program. It is developed through repeated physical activity and its goal is the ability to resist fatigue, thereby preventing fatigue-related injuries. Endurance training is at opposite ends of the spectrum from strength training. Whereas in the latter weight increases and repetitions decrease, in the former the emphasis is on increased repetitions combined with a reduction in weight.

Once optimal muscle and strength development has occurred, the athlete can reduce his workouts to two days per week, which is the minimal amount of time to maintain his level of strength.

Equipment

Good quality equipment, perfectly fitted, plays a very important part in injury prevention.[3] We will first consider the football helmet. The type of helmet selected depends upon the player who will be wearing it. The grade school player, as well as some high school players, does not require the amount of protection of older, larger athletes because the momentum generated by younger players is far less than that produced by the heavier and faster college and professional athletes. Since increased helmet protection adds weight and bulk, muscle fatigue will result when such a helmet is worn by a younger player with an underdeveloped neck. Other considerations in helmet selection include the shape of the player's head, his position on the team, his aggressiveness, and player performance.

The suspension helmet is the lightest but not always the most comfortable helmet. The padded-suspension helmet is more comfortable but it weighs more. The air helmet is a padded helmet that has air cells, which can be inflated after the helmet is on the player's head, to improve the fit and to possibly absorb low-intensity blows. The water helmet has compartments for liquid and is designed to afford greater protection from high-intensity blows. It is heavier than the other helmets and is intended only for the well-conditioned, more experienced athlete. The chin strap secures the helmet to the head by either two- or four-point attachments to the helmet. Four-point attachments are more effective in reducing helmet rocking. Regardless of the attachment used, all chinstraps must fit the chin snugly.

The face mask should consist of a bar frame covered with protective rubber. The choice of face mask style depends upon the position played. When fitting the mask, there must be no more than two finger widths between the mask and the chin or nose. When fitted properly, the face mask does not project out too far from the face and yet it is far enough away to avoid injury to the chin or mouth should the helmet rotate on the head during impact. Plastic loop fasteners on the face mask afford a convenient way of securing the face mask to the helmet, yet they can easily be cut off to remove the face mask from the helmet should an emergency arise.

Mouth protectors are required equipment for the prevention of dental injuries and in some instances of cerebral concussion.

Shoulder pad selection is determined by the position played. In general, the inner edge of the shoulder pad should be one-half inch from the neck. The clavicle and the deltoid regions must be protected with additional padding, which can be fastened to the shoulder to avoid dislodgement.

Any of the previously described pieces of equipment may be damaged with use, and each piece must be regularly inspected to make sure that all the parts are undamaged and still fit properly. Equipment check is the responsibility of each athlete.

MOVEMENT OF THE INJURED ATHLETE

The appropriate methods for treating on-field head and neck injuries were discussed in great detail in Chapters 9 and 10. We will focus our attention here on the proper way to take an injured player off the field and how to remove his equipment to permit examination.

Any player who is suspected to have suffered a head or neck injury must be removed from the field by litter *with his helmet left on!* In order to prevent doing further injury, moving the athlete onto the litter must be done gently, with no hurried movements. The first step in this process is to advise the athlete as to what is being done, requesting that he lie completely still and cooperate with the medical team. This step is essential because an injured player is a frightened player and, in this emotional state, it is not unlikely that he could resist efforts of the medical team to help him, thereby compounding his injuries. The next step is actually moving the player onto the fracture board. Although there are several methods the medical team can

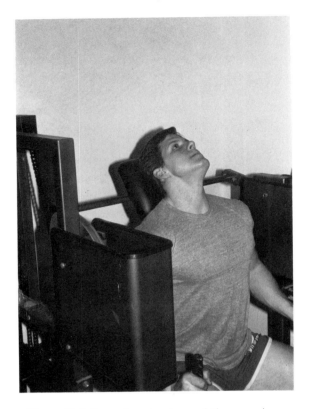

Figure 11-8. Isotonic extension resistive exercise.

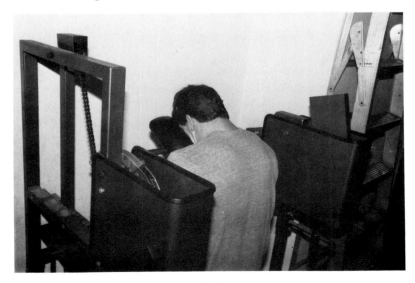

Figure 11-9. Isotonic flexion resistive exercise.

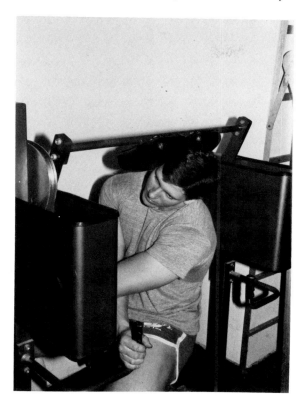

Figure 11-10. Isotonic lateral flexion resistive exercise.

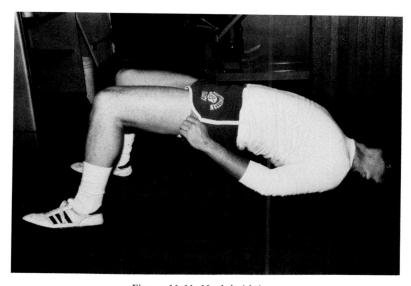

Figure 11-11. Neck bridging.

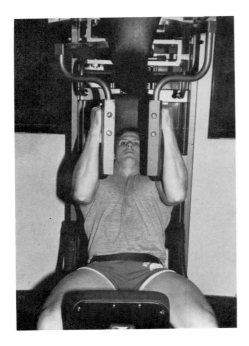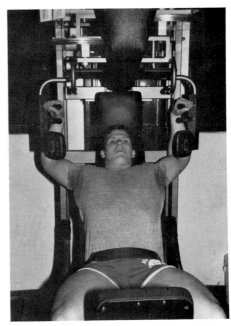

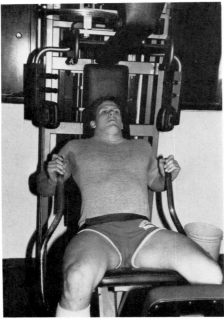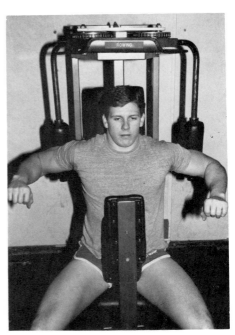

Figure 11-12. (Upper left) Fly exercise to develop pectoralis major and anterior deltoid muscles.

Figure 11-13. (Upper right) Fly exercise showing resistance encountered to reach final position.

Figure 11-14. (Lower left) Bench press. For pectoralis major muscle and triceps.

Figure 11-15. (Lower right) Rows. Rowing against resistance for posterior deltoid, rhomboids and trapezius muscle development.

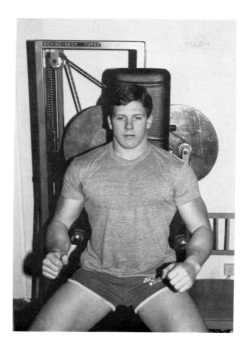

Figure 11-16. Behind neck torso for trapezius and latissumus dorsi muscles.

use to accomplish this, the safest and most efficient is the log-rolling technique. In this technique, there is one person in charge and he controls the player's head and neck. He positions his assistants as necessary so that the athlete's head, neck, and body will move as one unit onto the board. On command of the person in charge, the team rolls the athlete onto the board, where his head is then secured by either taping the helmet to the board with adhesive tape, or by sandbags, rolled up towels, or any other type of padding placed at both sides of his head to prevent head motion (Fig. 11-17).

Should the injured athlete develop difficulty breathing, it will be necessary to remove some of his equipment in order to permit access to his face. Two methods may be used to remove the face mask, the method being determined by the way the mask is attached to the helmet. In some instances, a bolt cutter will be required to cut off the mask (Fig. 11-18). Unfortunately, removing a mask with a bolt cutter is difficult, not to mention that this tool may not be immediately available. An easier removal method may be used if the face mask is mounted to the helmet by four or six plastic straps, since the straps can be cut with a pocket knife, scissors, or scalpel and the face mask removed from the helmet.

If it becomes absolutely essential that the helmet be removed from the head of an injured player before he reaches the hospital, a very strict and

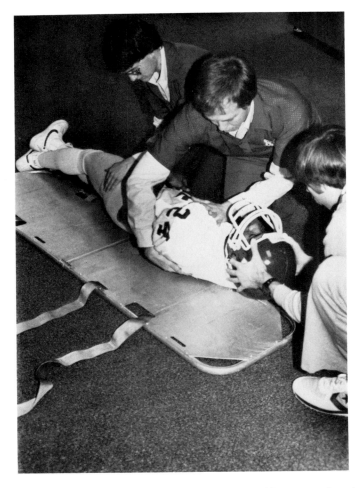

Figure 11-17. Log-rolling technique used to turn athlete with suspected neck fracture.

precise procedure must be followed.[7] First, the head and helmet are stabilized and the chinstrap is removed. This may be accomplished either by cutting the strap or by unsnapping it. The next step is to loosen the three snaps that hold each cheek pad in place by inserting a slender, flat object between the helmet and the cheek pad (Fig. 11-19). When the object is twisted slightly, the cheek pad will pop off. Slowly and gently the pads are slipped out from the space between the cheek and the helmet, making certain throughout the entire procedure that the helmet is securely held so that no movement is possible. Once both pads have been removed, the person holding the helmet prepares to ease the helmet off the athlete's head by placing his index fingers into the airholes of the helmet. A second person

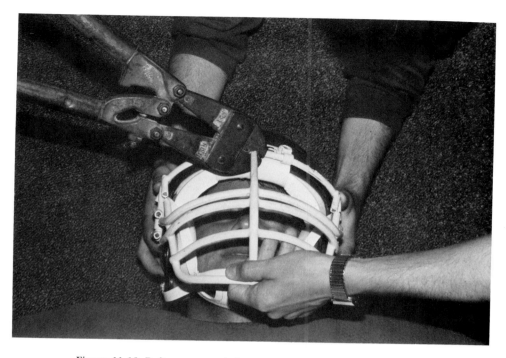

Figure 11-18. Bolt cutter needed to remove some types of face masks.

(ideally, a physician) positions his hands under the player's head and neck to support these structures as the helmet is slipped off the head (Fig. 11-20). After the helmet has been removed, sandbags are used to stabilize the head.

In order to carry out a thorough physical examination and to take x-rays, the shoulder pads must be removed. This procedure requires the assistance of several people. First the jersey is cut away from the shoulder pad. Next the shoulder pad lacing is cut. The straps that go under the arms and across the axillary region have to be detached from the front part of the shoulder pads and eventually cut away from the back part. If the athlete is wearing a neck collar or roll, their attachments must also be cut from the shoulder pads. Although there are very few neckrolls that attach to the helmet, care must be taken when removing the roll if it is attached in this manner. Once the neckroll has been removed, the athlete is then carefully rolled onto his side and the lacing of the shoulder pads in the back is cut. The deltoid pad of the shoulder pad is cut and removed. The athlete is then returned to the supine position and the remaining half of the shoulder pad is lifted off.

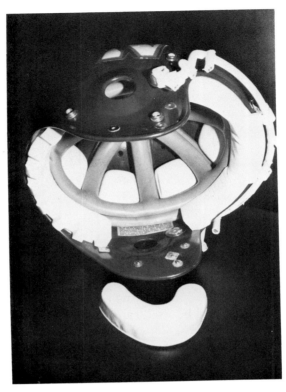

Figure 11-19. Removal of helmet in athlete with suspected neck injury. Remove cheek pads.

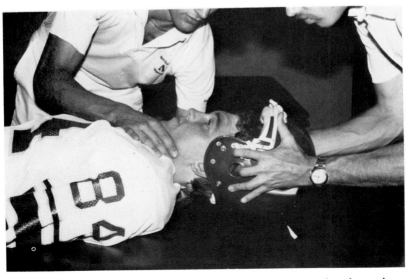

Figure 11-20. Carefully slide helmet off head while supporting the neck.

POST-INJURY REHABILITATION

Acute Phase

The primary modalities of treatment of the acute phase of head and neck injuries are ice, moist heat, ultrasound, and static or intermittent traction, and they may be used separately or in conjunction with one another. Ice is used to reduce muscle spasm, to help control possible bleeding from capillaries, and to provide an anesthetic effect. It can be administered either as an ice massage or in the form of cold packs. Ice is usually applied when the injury is not severe enough to require some type of immobilization and, depending upon the nature of the acute injury, it is applied for twenty-four to seventy-two hours.

Moist heat is a superficial form of heat that is used following the period of ice treatment. Moist heat helps to increase the circulation, relieve some of the soreness, and reduce spasm, allowing a greater range of motion of the injured area. Ultrasound is a method of applying heat to the deeper body tissues through the use of high-frequency sound waves, which are capable of being absorbed by some tissues, penetrating others, and merely reflecting off of others. This method should be used cautiously, however, and only when ordered by a physician, because nervous tissue, due to its protein content, can inadvertently be heated by ultrasound treatment, which can possibly result in nerve damage. Ultrasound, therefore, is contraindicated for use in the vicinity of the spinal cord. In many types of injuries, however, ultrasound can be very beneficial by producing heat in the deeper layers of tissue, thereby speeding up the recovery process. In such cases, it should be used daily for six minutes over a ten-day period.

Static and intermittent traction are appropriately used for some of the more chronic types of injuries, such as some nerve root injuries, brachial plexus stretches, or chronic sprains. Traction is not indicated for acute injuries, since it may aggravate such injuries. Moreover, injury that has caused a first, second, or third degree of strain of ligaments resulting in protective splinting through muscle spasm should not be treated by traction. When traction is used, it is important that the head and neck be placed in good postural alignment so that traction does not aggravate existing pain. Intermittent traction can provide some relief from pain when twenty seconds of traction is alternated with fifteen seconds of relaxation over a fifteen-minute period, one to two times per day, or in some cases every other day.

Reconditioning

Once the acute phase of the injury is over, the reconditioning process begins. This process is a slow one in which the injured part is exercised

gently but never to the point where movement becomes painful. Reconditioning exercises should be done five times a week until the injured part can
be moved painlessly through its full range of motion and muscle strength has
returned to its pre-injury level. For the purpose of our discussion, we will consider the reconditioning process of an athlete who has a chronic neck injury.

Chronic neck injuries require a program of strength-building exercises to
prevent the recurrence of such injuries. This program begins with passive
exercises performed five times a week until the athlete can move his neck
throughout its entire range of motion without pain. When this point is
reached, manual resistance should be applied, with the trainer's hand stabi-
lizing the athlete's shoulder girdle while he attempts to move his neck
throughout its range of motion. Three sets of ten range of motion exercises
should be done, with no more than a one- to one-and-one-half-minute break
between sets. Manual resistance will help to increase the athlete's range of
motion, strength, and endurance, but care must be taken not to increase the
number of repetitions or the amount of resistance too rapidly, since this
could cause additional injury or aggravate the present injury.

Once the athlete has progressed through a program of manual resistance,
he is probably ready for light Nautilus work performed under supervision.
Because the Nautilus itself has a certain amount of weight even without the
addition of weights, it may be that the machine may initially provide too
much resistance. Should this be the case, additional exercises performed
using manual resistance are indicated before Nautilus work can commence.
Once the athlete is strong enough to work out on the Nautilus machine, he
will follow the same program prescribed in our section on isotonic exercises.

The use of a cervical collar post-injury in order to prevent further injury
by restricting neck movement is not always advisable. Although the collar
does limit movement, it can also cause further injury by fixing one point of
the cervical spine, thereby causing excessive movement to occur at the area
just above the fixed level. This is potentially injurious, because the most
vulnerable point of an injured cervical spine is generally that area immediately above the level of limited flexibility, usually the C_5–C_6 level. In
addition, although ideally the collar should allow full range of physiologic
motion while restricting motion beyond this point, in actuality it is difficult
to accomplish this without also impairing normal motion. An example of
this problem occurred when we were fitting a lineman with a cervical collar
after he had received repeated brachial plexus injuries. When the athlete
was crouched in his offensive lineman stance, the collar restricted the extension of his neck so that he was unable to see above the knees of the opponent
in front of him (Fig. 11-21).

Many types of cervical collars are on the market today (Fig. 11-22). The
soft, round, sponge variety may allow free range of motion to occur while

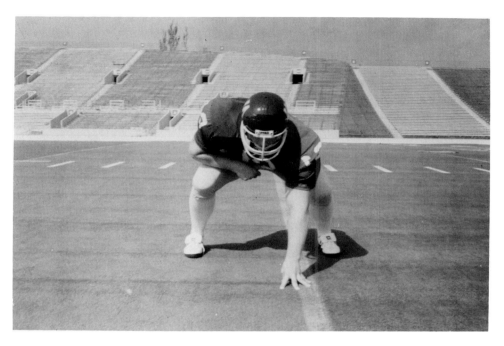

Figure 11-21. Shows limited vision of lineman when neck is restricted by collar.

stopping some of the extreme ranges of motion. These types of collars are often fastened to the shoulder pads so that the helmet impinges on the sides of the collar, preventing lateral motion. These collars do not, however, prevent neck rotation. Other types of collars project out further in an attempt to more effectively limit the range of motion. Some collars attach to the helmet and extend to the shoulder pads. Homemade collars can be devised using a hard or sponge core, with towels or additional sponge placed on the outside of the collar and attached to the shoulder pads. Homemade collars have the advantage of being custom fitted to meet the needs of a particular athlete, but it is nonetheless difficult to fashion a collar that will permit normal motion while restricting motion in the trauma range. Although many such devices have been developed, they have generally been unsuccessful.

When an athlete completes a program of post-injury rehabilitation, he still must pass several physical tests before he can return to competition. First, he must be able to move throughout the complete range of motion without pain. Secondly, he must have equal strength in all ranges of motion. Thirdly, there cannot be any muscle spasm in the cervical area or the shoulder girdle. Finally, there must be no pain, tingling, or numbness in the cervical region, shoulder girdle, or in any of the extremities. If all of these criteria are met, he may be fitted with his equipment and returned to active competition.

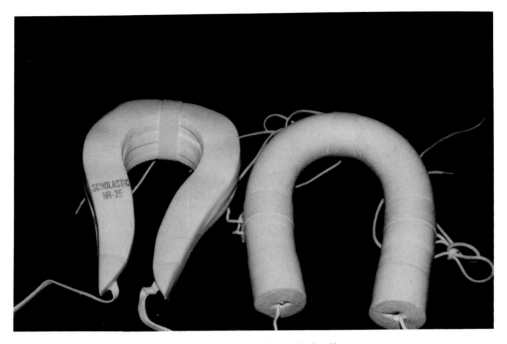

Figure 11-22. Types of cervical collars.

SUMMARY

Injuries are, unfortunately, a fairly common consequence of contact sports. This does not mean, however, that the numbers and seriousness of these injuries cannot be minimized by a concerted effort on the part of the players, coaches, and medical team toward a goal of injury prevention. Injury prevention begins with the team selection process, where only those players physically matched to the sport are chosen. Once selected, each player is expected to maintain peak physical and mental condition so that he is prepared to play in top form at all times. The purchase of the highest-quality equipment, individually fitted to the needs of each player, will also serve to prevent injuries. Finally, the coaching staff needs to stress injury prevention in training. When an injury does occur, proper on-field treatment can be an extremely important factor in preventing further injury as well as minimizing the effects of the injury. A carefully designed reconditioning program, initiated as soon as possible post-injury, will ensure that no athlete returns to the sport until he is once again in top playing condition.

REFERENCES

1. Albright J. P., Moses, J. M., Feldeck, H. G., Dolan, K. L., and Burmeister, L. F.: Non-fatal cervical spine injuries in interscholastic football. *JAMA, 236*:1243, 1976.
2. Beaulieu, J. A.: Developing a stretch program. *Physician & Sports Med, 9*:59, 1981.
3. Blasco, E. A.: A fit in time saves. *Selling Sporting Goods,* Sept:95, 1978, 95.
4. Hirata, I.: Conditioning and training of the competitive athlete. *J Sports Med, 1*:14, 1972.
5. Jensen, C. R., and Fisher, A. G.: *Scientific Basis of Athletic Conditioning.* Philadelphia, Lea & Febiger, 1972.
6. Klafs, C. E., and Arnheim, D. D.: *Modern Principles of Athletic Training,* 2nd Ed. St. Louis, Mosby, 1977.
7. Long, S. E., Reid, S. E., Sweeney, H. J., and Johnson, W. W.: Removing football helmets safely. *Physician & Sports Med, 8*:119, 1980.
8. Maroon, J., Kerin, T., Rehkopf, P., and McMaster, J.: A system for preventing athletic neck injuries. *Physician & Sports Med,* Oct:79, 1977.
9. O'Donoghue, D. H.: *Treatment of Injuries to Athletes,* 2nd Ed. Philadelphia, Saunders, 1970.
10. Sapega, A. A., Quedenfeld, T. C., Moyer, r. A., and Butler, R. A.: Biophysical factors in range of motion exercise. *Physician & Sports Med, 9*:57, 1981.

Chapter 12

SUGGESTIONS FOR SPORTS SAFETY

Sports safety must be of primary concern to everyone participating in any form of athletics. In this chapter, we will offer suggestions that can help to prevent injury and ensure the safety of participants in athletic activities.

The first requirement for promoting safety in sports is a complete physical examination for the potential athlete. This exam must focus first on any previous injuries. Should such old injuries exist, x-rays of the injury site must be taken to determine whether healing has been complete and if the individual is now fit to resume the sport. In addition, these x-rays become a permanent part of the athlete's record, to be referred to should any problems develop at a later date. In some instances, routine x-rays may be indicated, regardless of prior injuries. At the University of Iowa, cervical spine x-rays of the entering freshmen football team revealed that one-third had evidence of previous injury, although none was aware of such injury.

Abnormal tests or x-rays do not always mean the end of athletic activity, but some abnormal findings must be regarded as a red flag to further participation in contact sports. For example, during his entrance physical examination, a member of the incoming freshman football team at Northwestern University reported that he injured his neck two years earlier while playing high school football, when an opponent grasped his face mask and twisted his neck as he threw him to the ground. At the time of injury, his symptoms did not seem to warrant an extensive examination, and the boy continued to play without incident during the next two years. This past history of cervical injury was sufficient for us to order x-rays. The neck flexion films revealed a 9 to 11 millimeter anterior dislocation of the cervical spine at the C_1–C_2 junction (Figs. 12-1 & 12-2),[3] which was reduced when the neck was extended (Fig. 12-3). Although there was no evidence of neurologic deficit, the joint was unstable due to the torn ligaments, and the boy was dropped from the team. Similarly, a football player who has a history of repeated concussions, but who has no gross neurologic deficit, must be encouraged to switch to a non-contact sport, to reduce the likelihood of serious head injury resulting from the cumulative effects of repeated blows.

The absence of one of a pair of organs, such as kidneys, testes, or ovaries, does not automatically mean exclusion from contact sports, provided the remaining organ can be protected. A missing or blind eye, however, is an

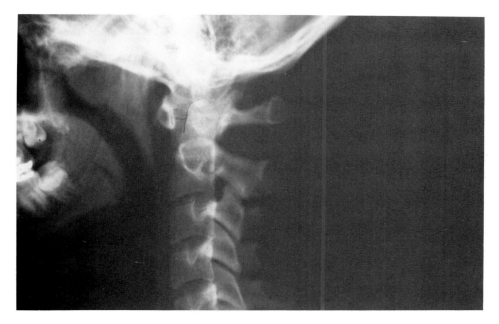

Figure 12-1. Cervical spine x-ray examination in flexion shows increased space between the anterior arch of C_1 and the odontoid process of C_2.

entirely different situation. Although protective goggles can be fitted to prevent injury to the remaining eye, absence of vision on one side of the body places the athlete in jeopardy. He would be unable to anticipate a blow to his blind side and, therefore, could not protect himself from injury. The high potential for injury to a partially sighted participant in contact sports must be seriously considered, with each case evaluated individually. Several one-eyed athletes have, it must be noted, experienced virtually no problems related to their partial sightedness, and we have had a partially sighted player on the Northwestern football team. In that situation we notified the athlete and his parents of the additional risk of injury. All of them were required to advise us in writing that they had been apprised of the dangers and were willing to accept any associated risks so that the athlete could continue to play. A letter of consent does not, of course, relieve the school of responsibility for care of a subsequently injured athlete, but it does serve to protect the school from unnecessary criticism.

Proper conditioning is the second requirement for maximizing sports safety. Conditioning is a gradual process where physical effort is slowly increased as the individual's endurance builds. Once optimal conditioning has been achieved, the athlete must maintain this condition throughout the playing season, and between seasons as well. No out-of-condition athlete

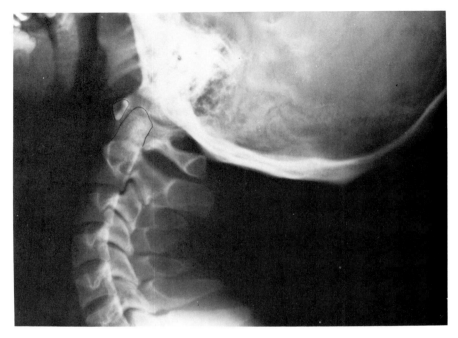

Figure 12-2. X-ray of the cervical spine in extension shows the odontoid process moved anteriorly to its near-normal position.

should be permitted to participate until he gets back into top shape. Conditioning methods have been discussed in detail in Chapter 11, but, obviously, each type of sport requires its own specific conditioning exercises.

With regard to football, proper positioning plays a significant role in promoting safety on the field. The safest position for the athlete's head and neck is one that allows him to see an oncoming impact. To accomplish this, the neck must be in a neutral or slightly extended position, enabling the player to see and adjust to any movement of his opponent (Fig. 12-4). In this position, the neck muscles can offer maximum resistance to any forced extension. Moreover, the athlete can also use his arms and shoulders to tackle and block, thereby avoiding a direct hit. Positioning techniques must be demonstrated by the coach to the team, so that both player performance and safety can be improved.

Grouping players according to their age, size, and ability is another means of increasing sports safety. Younger and smaller players are unprepared for and physically underdeveloped to handle the hard body blows associated with contact sports such as football.[1] A few years of physical growth and experience combined with specific conditioning programs will help to prepare a player for a more intense, hard-hitting game. It is not unusual,

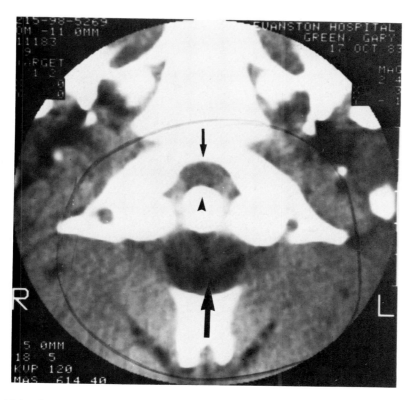

Figure 12-3. The CAT scan of the cervical spine shows the odontoid process (middle arrow) of C_2 dislocated posteriorly to increase the interval between it and the anterior arch of C_1 (upper arrow) and to make intimate contact with the spinal cord (lower arrow). This indicates that the very strong transverse ligament extending from each lateral mass of C_1 behind the odontoid process has been torn. The alar ligaments anterior-lateral to the odontoid process are seen.

however, for a star high school athlete to be shaken up by the blows received during his first few college games. Coaches must recognize this problem and work with their new players, so that these new members of the team will be both mentally and physically equipped to participate in a stepped-up game.

The mental attitude of the athlete plays a key role in insuring his safety in sports participation. Both the motivation to play and the recognition of a sport's inherent risks are primary components in the development of a good mental attitude. Either extreme of under- or over-motivation can predispose a player to injury. The motivation of a player can be undermined by a poor team record or even by losing a particular game. In this situation, minor injuries incurred assume major proportions as the player tries to avoid further participation. Another factor contributing to decreased motivation is the worry of an injured but now recovered athlete that he will re-injure

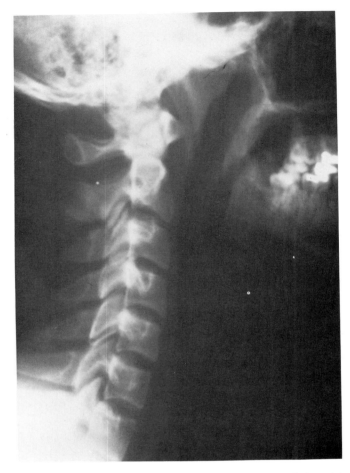

Figure 12-4. X-ray view of the neck in its normal, slightly extended position. Courtesy of Appleteon-Century-Crofts.

himself. This fear can result in a favoring of the injured area and a dimin-ished enthusiasm for the sport. Similarly, seeing a teammate receiving an injury may cause an athlete to worry about being injured himself. Ironically, as this player becomes over-cautious in an attempt to protect himself from injury, the likelihood of his actually being injured increases. Clearly, then, any player who lacks a strong desire to participate in a sport should not play.

The highly motivated athlete is also at risk for injury. Such a player may receive an injury and yet not report it, particularly when he is a member of a winning team or when competition for his position is keen. Other overly motivated athletes take unnecessary risks, refusing to recognize the injury potential for their actions. In these instances, the motivation to play has been carried to the extreme, and, like his under-motivated counterpart, the over-motivated player is vulnerable to injury. Coaches must recognize this danger and try to temper over-enthusiasm in their players in order to ensure their safety.

The elimination of unsportsmanlike conduct is another requirement for promoting sports safety. Intentional attempts to injure an opponent may actually cause injury to both the offensive and defensive player. Nowhere is this more apparent than in the illegal practice of spearing, where a player intentionally drives the dome of his helmet into his opponent. Injuries to the hands or ribs of the opponent are generally mild and secondary to the injury potential to the spearing player himself. Complete paralysis or sudden death is not an unlikely consequence of this illegal action, as the rising number of such injuries demonstrates. Players must understand that spearing literally endangers their lives, and coaches must neither teach nor permit spearing or other illegal tactics. Finally, game officials must be diligent in their responsibility to penalize any offenders.

It is crucial that, as a sport develops and changes, the rules are modified to keep pace. The National Federation of State High Schools Associations Rules Committee and the NCAA Football Rules Committee have made many such rule revisions over the years. Most rules in contact sports are intended to protect the athlete from an unexpected blow, such as tackling an athlete who is out-of-bounds, or after the referee's whistle signals the end of the play, or once the quarterback has thrown the ball and is watching it travel. Again, it is up to the players, coaches, and officials to see that all rules are strictly followed, with all violations penalized.

In the case of football and other team contact sports, the team physician plays a major role in promoting sport safety. He must combine his knowledge of medicine with motivational psychology and a thorough understanding of the sport in order to function effectively. Because the team physician believes in the benefits of the sport, he will not underestimate the importance of playing to an athlete, and any decision to remove a player from the game will not be made lightly.

It is the team physician who is responsible for any decision concerning the length of time an injured player must remain on the sidelines. This decision cannot be influenced by the wishes of the athlete, coach, parents, or spectators but must be made on the basis of medical judgment, experience, and careful observation of the player. The only way a team doctor can make such decisions is if he is actually *on the sidelines,* watching each play of the game, and calling the player off the field if the doctor feels an injury may have occurred. The team physician must combine a psychological examination with a physical examination in order to completely evaluate a possible injury. The speed with which an athlete can be returned to the game depends on several variables, the first of which is, obviously, the seriousness of the injury. Head and neck injuries are potentially catastrophic and must be thoroughly evaluated before returning the athlete to the game, whereupon he must be closely observed for any signs of disability.

The second variable determining whether an injured player can return to the game is the motivation of the athlete himself. Some players recover very quickly, others take longer. In no case should a player be returned to the game against his wishes.

The physical condition of a player before injury is another determining factor as to when he may return to the game. A healthy, well-conditioned athlete may suffer little damage from a hard hit, while his previously injured teammate could be seriously injured by a similar blow.

Cooperation on the part of the player, coach, and trainer is the final variable in the matter of when an injured athlete may resume play. The player must follow the instructions of the team physician, reporting for all treatment appointments, and avoiding any forbidden activity. The coach must make certain that the player cooperates with the instructions of the team doctor. Furthermore, the coach must not put undue pressure on the doctor regarding the availability of the player, nor put him back in the game without the doctor's approval. The trainer, in his capacity as assistant to the team physician, is primarily responsible for reconditioning the injured athlete. Because of the importance of this position, the National Athletic Trainers Association has established standardized requirements for team trainers. These include 1800 hours of practical experience under the guidance of a certified trainer, a college degree or a degree in physical therapy, and qualification in cardiopulmonary resuscitation. An effective trainer establishes a good relationship with the players, so that they feel free to come to him concerning potential injuries and other training problems. The trainer cannot dispense drugs on his own but must consult with the team physician, who will prescribe if necessary. The trainer must also keep accurate records of all dispensed drugs. In addition, he needs to be acutely aware of injury prevention, both to players and spectators alike, such as those people who watch the game from the sidelines and who risk collision with a player running out-of-bounds.

Many suggestions have been given to improve the safety features of athletic equipment. To avoid injury to the neck it was suggested that the helmet should be tethered to the shoulder pads so as to avoid fracture or dislocation of the neck as the neck is driven into the trauma range of motion. It has been shown that a rigid neck is much more vulnerable to injury than a well-developed one that is allowed to move at will.[2,4] Restricting the neck would cut down on the athlete's maneuverability and cause more injuries. Some athletes feel that bushy hair on their heads offers a good energy-absorbing effect and that they would be unwilling to cut their hair because of this feature. The specifications of the helmet is that it must fit properly. When the helmet is fitted to dry hair, it is normally snug; but after strenuous exercise, when the hair gets wet, the helmet can become quite loose. The face mask was added to prevent injury to the face, but it soon became apparent that this addition puts the neck into very serious jeopardy. We cannot remove the face mask and allow face injuries to recur, so the rules against grasping a face mask and whipping the head must be rigidly enforced.

SUMMARY

While there will always be some injuries associated with football and other contact sports, it is the obligation of everyone involved in these sports to minimize the incidence and severity of such injuries. To accomplish this goal, we recommend complete physical examinations at the start of each season for all new players and annual checkups for returning athletes. Any abnormalities in these examinations must be thoroughly evaluated before an individual is pronounced fit to play. Once this determination has been made, an intensive conditioning program will help to keep the team members in top condition, thereby increasing their chances of remaining injury-free, particularly when they observe proper positioning techniques. Obviously, another key factor in reducing injuries is grouping players according to their age, size, and ability.

The mental attitude of the athlete plays a significant role in ensuring his safety. Both extremes of high and low motivation carry with them the increased risk of injury. Unsportsmanlike conduct, including illegal actions such as spearing, is a major cause of sports injuries. It must be emphatically prohibited by coaches and consistently penalized by officials. Similarly, rule changes are often necessary as a sport develops, and these changes help to promote sports safety.

Finally, in a situation where an injury has occurred, its seriousness can be minimized when the player, coach, and trainer follow the treatment program designed by the team physician, who must be ultimately responsible for all decisions concerning the degree of injury and the ability of the athlete to play.

REFERENCES

1. Culver, R. H., Bender, M., and Melvin, J. W.: Mechanisms, tolerances and responses obtained under dynamic superior-inferior impacts. University of Michigan Highway Safety Research Institute, 78-21, May, 1978.
2. Ommaya, A. K., Hirsch, A. E., Flamm, E. S., and Mahone, R. M.: Cerebral concussion in the monkey: An experimental model. *Science, 153*(3732): 211, July, 1966.
3. Torg, J. S.: *Athletic Injuries of the Head, Neck and Face.* Philadelphia, Lea & Febiger, 1982, pp. 130 and 176.
4. White, R. J., and Albin, M. S.: Spine and spinal cord injury. In Gurdjian, E. S. et al. (Ed.): *Impact Injury and Crash Protection.* Springfield, Thomas, 1970, p. 63.

INDEX